Practical Procedures in Acute Emergency Medicine

To our Families

Practical Procedures in Accident and Emergency Medicine

David G Ferguson FRCS (Edin.)

Consultant in Accident and Emergency Medicine, Royal Hallamshire
Hospital, Sheffield

Stuart M Lord FRCS (Glasg.)

Consultant in Accident and Emergency Medicine, Royal Liverpool
Hospital

Butterworths

London ● Boston ● Durban ● Singapore ● Sydney ● Toronto ● Wellington

First published, 1986

© Butterworth & Co. (Publishers) Ltd, 1986

British Library Cataloguing in Publication Data

Ferguson, David G.
    Practical procedures in accident and
    emergency medicine.
    1. Emergency medicine
    I. Title.   II. Lord, Stuart M.
    616'.025   RC86.7

    ISBN 0-407-00360-6

Library of Congress Cataloging in Publication Data

Ferguson, David G.
    Practical procedures in accident and
emergency medicine.

    Includes index.
    1. Emergency medicine   2. Wounds and injuries –
Treatment.   I. Lord, Stuart M.   II. Title.
[DNLM: 1. Accidents. 2. Emergencies. 3. Emergency
Medicine – methods. WB 105 F352p]
RC86.7.F47   1986   616'.025   85-31357

    ISBN 0-407-00360-6

Photoset by Butterworths Litho Preparation Department
Printed and bound in Great Britain by
Robert Hartnoll (1985) Limited, Bodmin, Cornwall

Preface

This book has been written primarily for senior medical students and newly qualified doctors but it is hoped other doctors and associated staff may find it useful. The authors know that there are other ways of undertaking many of the procedures listed but those methods described have been found to be effective.

Each procedure is described in text on the left hand page with relevant drawings on the right hand page. There are only a few double pages of text, mainly in the introduction to some sections. Wherever possible the text has been laid out to show: (1) title of procedure; (2) the use of the procedure; (3) equipment required (lines prefixed with letters); (4) the procedure itself; and (5) significant complications of the procedure.

We wish to thank particularly Patrick Elliott who has prepared all the drawings and without whose talent we could not have produced the book.

The following diagrams are reproduced by kind permission of Churchill Livingstone: p. 7 is taken from *The Illustrated Guide to Surgical Practice* by J. Freidin and V. Marshall, p. 3, 1984; p. 39 from *Fundamental Techniques of Plastic Surgery and Their Surgical Applications* by I. A. McGregor, 1975; pp. 185, 199 from *The Closed Treatment of Common Fractures* by J. Charnley, 1970; and p. 199 from *Outline of Fractures* by J. Crawford Adams, 1976.

David G. Ferguson
Stuart M. Lord

Contents

Section 4 Cardiac procedures

Section 5 Abdominal procedures

Section 6 Local anaesthetic

Section 7   Minor Surgical Procedures

Section 8   Bones and joints

Section 9 ENT, Eyes and Dentistry

Section 10 Foreign Bodies

Section 1
Basic principles

1 Scrubbing up

This is the washing of hands and forearms for the carrying out of sterile procedures

A   Warm water
B   Soap or scrubbing up liquid, such as Chlorhexidine or Betadine
C   Nail brush
D   Socially clean hands with neat short nails

1   Adjust the water temperature to suit you. The water may have to run for a while to allow the hot water to 'arrive'. It is worth waiting a few minutes for this.
2   Roll up your sleeves so that they stay up. They should be rolled above the elbow. Remove rings, watches and bracelets etc.
3   Wet both hands and forearms and apply an elbow to the scrub-up fluid dispenser (**a**). Collect a few drops of the fluid in the palm of the hand and then apply to the hands and forearms, or alternatively use a bar of soap.
4   Wash around the fingers and thumb, and then around the hands and up the forearms to the elbows.
5   Take a sterile nail brush which will have to be opened and given to you, or removed from a sterile dispenser by applying an elbow to the lever.
6   Scrub around and under the nails and then give a light scrub to the palms of the hands and the fingers (**b**). There is no need to carry this out to excess, as it only tends to 'dig up' more organisms from various skin crevices.
7   Wash down the hands and the elbows, keeping the hands up so that the water runs down from the hands to the elbows.
8   Repeat the scrub as above. In all take some 5 minutes.
9   When you have finished, keep the hands in the air, above the level of the elbows and turn off the taps with your elbows.
10   Take a sterile towel and dry both hands well, still keeping them up so that any drips run off the elbows. If the hands are not well dried, it is difficult to put surgical gloves on.
11   Take the towel in one hand and carefully draw it from the wrist towards the elbow, so as to dry the forearm (**c**). Do not go beyond the area that was scrubbed, which means leaving a small undried area of the forearm at the elbow. Carefully take the towel in the other hand so as not to touch the part which was used to dry the first forearm, and with a fresh area of towel repeat the drying manoeuvre on the other forearm.
12   Keep your hands up in front of you and do not touch anything.

1   Scrubbing up

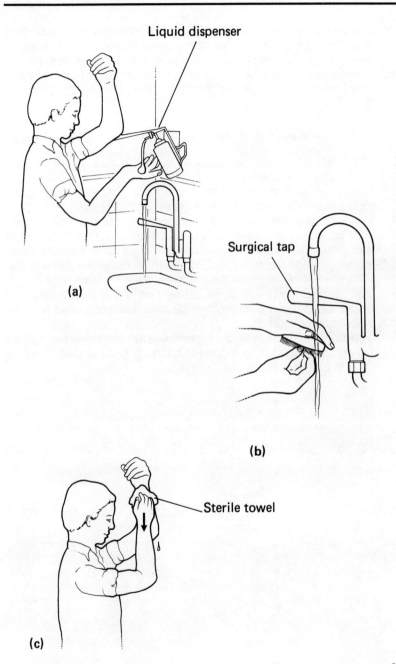

Liquid dispenser

(a)

Surgical tap

(b)

Sterile towel

(c)

2 Gloving up

Gloves come in various forms. There is a tendency in the Accident and Emergency Department to use the thinner, less expensive gloves for minor procedures such as suturing. The gloves used in theatre are more robust, and they come in a full range of hand sizes, whereas the cheaper gloves may only be available as small, medium or large.

A   Sterile glove pack of appropriate size for you

1   The basic rule is that the outside of the glove must not be touched by an ungloved hand.
2   The outer pack is opened by a nurse who drops the inner pack onto a sterile surface, such as an open basic dressing pack.
3   Open out the inner pack, taking care not to touch the gloves (**a**).
4   Pick up the upper folded edge of the left glove with the right hand and slip the left hand into the glove (**b**). The thumb of the left hand, which is inside the glove, should catch the rim of the glove so the folded edge of the glove does not slip back too soon (**c**).
5   The left hand with the glove partially on it can then be slipped under the fold of the right glove (**d**), which is then pulled onto the right hand (**e**) and (**f**).
6   The right hand can then go under the edge of the left-hand glove (**g**) and so pull it fully onto the left hand, allowing the left thumb to go into its glove thumb (**h**).

4

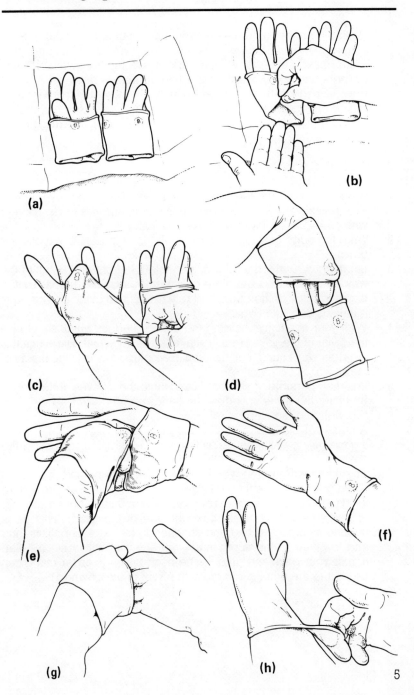

3 Gowning up

To enter an operating theatre, you must change from your outside clothes to theatre clothes and boots. When you are in the changing room, make sure that all the various articles are available, i.e., trousers and a top, mask and a hat. Is there a draw-cord in the trousers and are they of an acceptable size for you. If there is some article missing, ask for it.

When in theatre, you will have to gown up if you are going to assist.

A A surgical gown of the correct size

1 After scrubbing up, the gown pack is opened for you by a nurse. This reveals an inner pack which is sterile and has to be opened with care. Do not touch the outer covering.

2 Take the edge of the pack and gently draw it open to expose the gown.

3 Lift the gown, which is folded, and hold it in front of you, out of the way of trolleys and people etc. Hold it at shoulder height by the exposed edge of the gown, and release the rest of the gown so that it unfolds in front of you.

4 With your hands just holding the exposed edge, which should be the collar of the gown, gently shake the gown to make sure that it is the right way round, i.e., that you are looking towards the inside of the gown.

5 It is then possible to slip both hands into the sleeves of the gown. By lifting the arms upwards, the hands and the arms should then slip well into the sleeves (**a**).

6 A nurse will stand behind you and pull the gown onto you. It takes a good pull to push the hands through the elasticated wrists of the gown.

7 The nurse will then tie you into the gown from behind (**b**).

8 Some gowns have a flap to protect the back area. The procedure for tying this flap is only carried out after you have put on surgical gloves. There is a tie at the right side of the gown. This tie is undone, one end is long and attached to the back flap. This long end is given to the scrub nurse (**c**) and she will draw the flap across your back and give the tie back to you in order that it can be tied to the other end across the front of the gown (**d**).

3 Gowning up

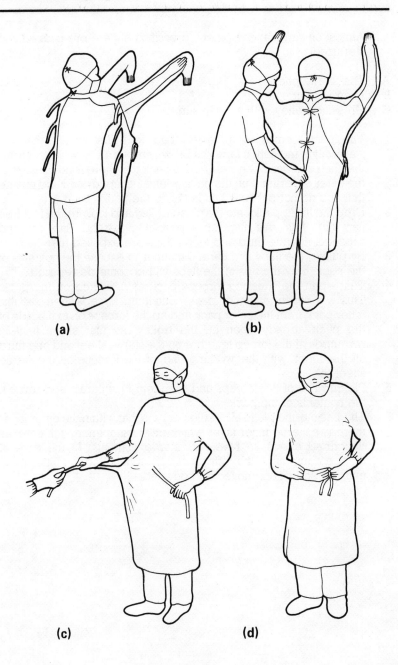

(a)

(b)

(c)

(d)

7

4 Opening sterile packs

Almost all surgical equipment, dressings etc are pre-packed and sterilized.

A   The sterile pack
B   Dressing forceps
C   Dressing trolley with a clean surface

1   The pack comes in a sealed bag (**a**). First check that the sterilization indication tape has brown stripes on it, which confirms that the pack has been sterilized. Check that there is no damage to the outer covering. Pull the pack open at its upper end and ensure that you do not put your hands inside the pack.

2   Drop the inner pack onto the clean trolley and look for the first free flap (**b**). Pull this flap to expose the second flap (**c**) and subsequently the third and fourth flaps are exposed (**d**).

3   By pulling the flaps in a careful manner to expose the contents of the pack, only the tips of the flaps will become desterilized.

4   Tear open the dressing forceps pack as indicated on the pack. This will reveal an inner pack containing forceps. Remove this inner pack from the outer pack and tip the forceps on to the side of the pack already open on the trolley, so that approximately two-thirds of the forcep length is on the sterile sheet and one-third off the sheet, with the 'working end' of the forceps on the sterile sheet (**e**).

5   Pick up two of the forceps and use them to separate and sort out the contents of the pack.

6   The basic principle to all sterile packs is that within the outer layer there is a sterile inner layer which must be opened with care, as described above, to reveal its sterile contents. In the case of theatre equipment, the individual who is handling the inner pack must be scrubbed, gloved and gowned.

4 Opening sterile packs

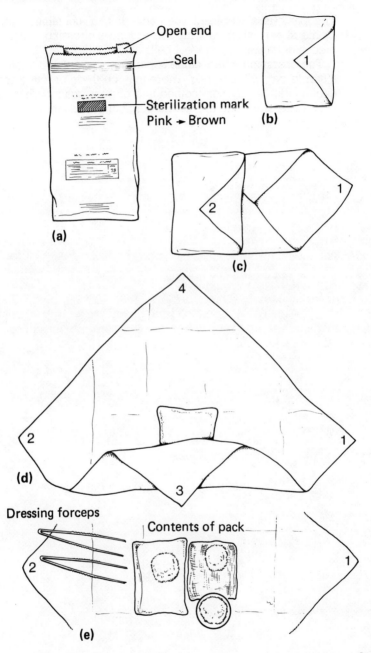

Open end

Seal

Sterilization mark
Pink → Brown

(a)

(b)

(c)

(d)

Dressing forceps

Contents of pack

(e)

5 Contents of basic dressing pack

The pack is a sterilized pre-packed 'bag' containing an inner sterile sheet, which is wrapped around a dressing towel, a few pieces of gauze, cotton wool balls and a gallipot.

The dressing forceps come separately packed and again are in a sterile bag within a bag. There may be three or four forceps in each pack, usually non-toothed and of poor quality. They are for use in dressings and are not for surgical procedures.

5 Contents of basic dressing pack

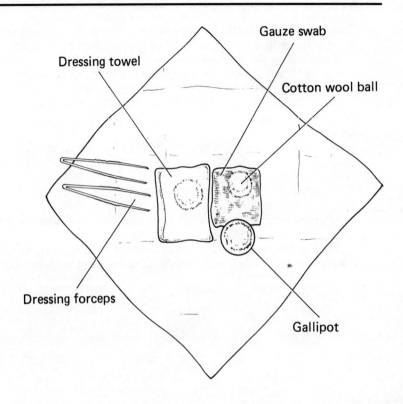

Gauze swab

Dressing towel

Cotton wool ball

Dressing forceps

Gallipot

6 Contents of suture pack

This will differ from department to department. It may come in a plastic tray with 'built in' gallipots or it may come in a cardboard tray containing the instruments only.

The pack will contain needleholders. These will be straight or curved. They have a ratchet mechanism to lock the needle in position. Some departments may use Gillies forceps which do not have a ratchet lock and have scissor edges incorporated in the forceps.

There will be a pair of toothed forceps for gently handling the skin, and maybe a pair of non-toothed forceps for removing foreign bodies and wound exploration.

Mosquito forceps are usually included for controlling small bleeding points and for clipping sutures before they are tied.

Suture scissors are included for cutting sutures. They are no good for cutting other materials or tissues.

Some units have a 'plastic surgical pack' which contains finer instruments and skin hooks. This is used for fine cosmetic work.

6 Contents of suture pack

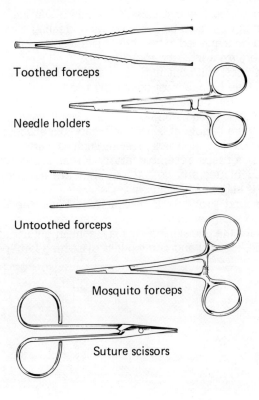

Toothed forceps

Needle holders

Untoothed forceps

Mosquito forceps

Suture scissors

7 Contents of incision pack

This contains the instruments for minor surgical procedures. It should not be used as a quick way of dealing with problems that should be managed in the accident and emergency theatre, which may require a little more organizing.

The pack will contain a No. 3 scalpel handle with or without a blade. The blades most commonly used are a No. 10, the smaller No. 15, or the pointed No. 11.

A curette (Volkmann's Spoon) is a small spoon with sharpened edges on a handle. It is used to scrape out abscess cavities or for the removal of superficial lesions such as warts.

Sinus forceps resemble artery forceps, but have long blunt pointed blades and no ratchet. They are used to explore small wounds and wound sinuses.

A wound probe looks like a large blunt needle and it is for probing small wounds or abscess cavities.

Finally the incision pack may contain suture scissors, artery forceps, toothed and non-toothed dissecting forceps.

7 Contents of incision pack

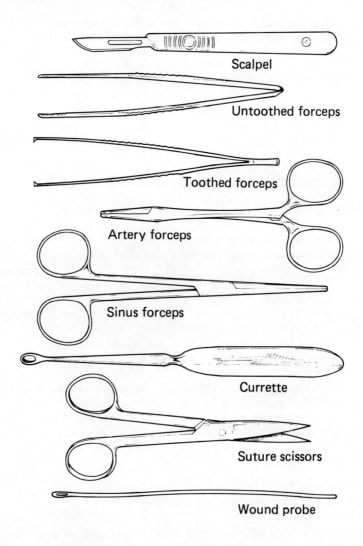

Scalpel

Untoothed forceps

Toothed forceps

Artery forceps

Sinus forceps

Currette

Suture scissors

Wound probe

8 Cleaning solutions

These are solutions used to generally clean wounds and remove foreign matter. They are also often antiseptic.

Desired properties of cleaning solutions

1 Non-irritant to the skin and wound
2 Detergent if possible
3 Antiseptic

Commonly used cleaning solutions

A Soap and water is often forgotten. The patient can wash around his own wound without causing himself undue discomfort and he can clean off a lot of dirt including industrial grime.
B Swarfega is excellent for removing oily materials.
C Normal saline comes either in 500 ml bottles or in sachets. It is cheap but has no particular advantages.
D Chlorhexidine is a skin disinfectant with detergent properties. It comes in many proprietary preparations, e.g., Savlodil, Savlon and Hibitane.
E Alcohol tends to sting the wound. It is generally used to clean skin around injection sites, or to dry the skin before applying dressings.
F Hydrogen peroxide is used in a 3 per cent solution (10 volumes). It is very good for cleaning wounds, as it tends to bubble and lift out debris. It is also useful for deodorizing infected wounds.
G Iodine compounds. First check that the patient does not have an iodine sensitivity. These compounds can come as scrub-up solutions, or in alcohol based solutions. They can be used for skin preparation.

Basic uses of cleaning solutions

1 For the general cleaning of wounds use Chlorhexidine solution or normal saline.
2 For the cleaning of deep contaminated wounds and leg ulcers, use hydrogen peroxide.
3 For skin preparation for minor surgical procedures, use a solution containing a dye, such as Hibitane or an iodine solution. The area which has been cleaned can then be clearly seen and defined, reducing the chances of contamination.

8 Cleaning solutions

4   When a patient has a particularly contaminated wound, such as can occur from industrial grime, let him wash the area himself with soap and water or with Swarfega.

9 Dressings

Dry dressings

These can be used to give protection to a wound which has dried and scabbed over, but which still needs to be covered. They are often used to give increased absorbency for exudates, but when this is done they should be placed over a non-adherent dressing, as they tend to become stuck down to the wounds and then are very uncomfortable to remove.

A Gauze is a loose woven cotton material, routinely used to clean wounds and as a dry dressing.
B Gamgee consists of thick layers of absorbent cotton between two layers of absorbent gauze. It is very good for heavy exudates or it can be used to dress wounds where there is heavy bleeding.
C Pressure dressings are most readily made from a wad of gauze applied directly to a wound and then held in place by a crepe bandage.

Non-adherent dressings

These are absorbent dressings, such as cotton, which are covered with a non-adherent layer. This layer differs in different proprietary dressings.

They are applied directly to the wound, and they absorb exudate and keep the wound relatively dry. They should not adhere to the wound.

They come in pre-wrapped packages of various sizes. The packet is torn open and its contents should be dropped on to an open dressing pack. Check which side of the dressing is non-adherent, it is usually shiny and looks like cellophane. The dressing should be picked up with forceps and placed on the already cleaned wound and held in place by some adhesive tape.

Impregnated gauze

These are layers of gauze, impregnated with soft paraffin. Many of the preparations contain an antiseptic or antibiotic. It is doubtful if there is any advantage in using those preparations containing an antibiotic, and there are certainly disadvantages in doing so.

18

9 Dressings

They are used to cover raw surfaces such as deep abrasions or an area of total skin loss, such as in a pretibial laceration.

The impregnated gauze (tulle gras) can come either as pre-packed individual pieces ($10 \times 10\,cm$) or in a box containing many metres of the gauze. When the individual pack is opened the tulle gras should be dropped on to an open dressing pack. The greaseproof paper will have to be peeled off one side. Cut and/or fold the tulle gras to size and remove the other paper. Apply the tulle gras to the wound with dressing forceps. Cover with another dressing such as gauze.

If tulle gras is used as a 'wick', pick the piece up by its centre and make this the tip of the wick. This means that the free edges which tend to fray will be outside the wound, so there will be less chance of a small piece of cotton being left in the wound.

10 Handling instruments

Most surgical instruments are made for right-handed people and they require practice to use them properly.

Scissors

These are made in such a way, that as they are held in the right hand, the blades are forced together and this increases the cutting ability. If they are held in the left hand, this does not occur.

Place the right thumb in the (L) loop and the right ring finger in the (R) loop. The right index finger then rests on the screw holding the blades together, and the right middle finger rests alongside the right leg of the scissors. The scissors can then be steadied and used for fine work.

Needleholders

These are held just like scissors but there is also a ratchet to be controlled. To close the ratchet just squeeze the limbs together. The problem is unlocking the ratchet, which is achieved with the right index and middle fingers laid alongside the (R) loop. Because the ratchet has the (R) limb on the top of the (L) limb pushing with the thumb against the pull of the other fingers unlocks the ratchet.

If the needleholders are curved, they are held so that the curve is away from the fingers, bringing the tip of the instrument closer to the patient.

Forceps

These are held like a pen. The index finger rests along one limb and the thumb rests along the other limb. The natural spring of the instrument, which keeps them open, gives the necessary resistance to hold them.

Forceps should always be used gently as they will crush tissues. Toothed forceps should be used on skin as they can steady the skin edge with less pressure than non-toothed forceps.

10 Handling instruments

Scissors

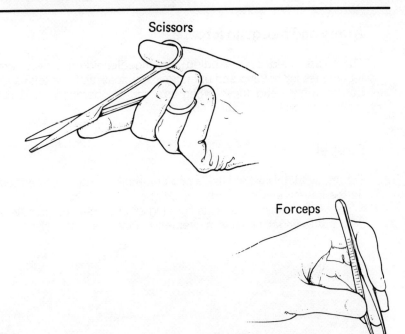

Forceps

Needle holder

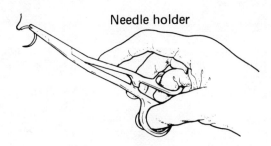

10 Handling instruments

Artery and mosquito forceps

These are held and handled like needleholders. There are techniques for holding and opening instruments with the left hand, but you only need these when assisting at operations, and the techniques will be taught then.

Scalpel

For fine work this is held like a pen or pencil and the hand can rest on the patient and so steady the point of the scalpel.

For larger incisions such as opening an abdomen, the handle is held in the finger tips and movements come from the wrist.

10 Handling instruments

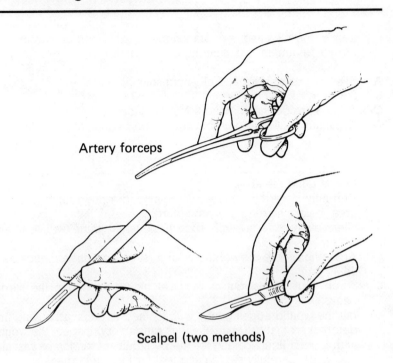

Artery forceps

Scalpel (two methods)

11 Wound toilet

This is the cleaning, exploration and preparation of a wound for further treatment, e.g. suturing or dressing.

A   Basic dressing pack and cleaning solution
B   Suture pack
C   A No. 3 scalpel handle and a No. 10 blade
D   Local anaesthetic. 1 per cent lignocaine, syringe and needle. (*See page 142*)

1   Obtain a good exposure of the wound by removing any clothing from around the area.
2   Carefully determine nerve, vascular and tendon function in the area, before starting any procedure.
3   Clean away excessive dirt, such as industrial grime, with soap and water.
4   Anaesthetize the area of the wound (*see Local anaesthetics page 142*)
5   Scrub your hands, put on surgical gloves and open the sterile packs.
6   Lift the wound edges gently with toothed forceps (**a**), having first determined that the anaesthetic is satisfactory. Inspect the wound with a good light, looking for the possibility of tendon or vascular injury (**b**). Carefully search and feel for foreign bodies.
7   Gently clean the inner aspect of the wound with gauze. If it is a deep wound, probe the wound to gain an idea of its size and direction. Use forceps to gently open the depths of the wound to give a better view. A syringe fitted with a needle and filled with normal saline can be used to flush foreign material from the wound.
8   Bleeding can be troublesome. Apply pressure to each side of the wound with your fingers and see if that controls the problem. If a definite bleeding point can be identified, apply a mosquito forcep to it. When the bleeding is persistent and it is obscuring everything, apply pressure directly to the wound and wait for five minutes. In a situation where the wound is in a limb, a sphygmomanometer cuff can be applied proximal to the wound and the pressure in the cuff raised to 200 mm Hg. This is uncomfortable for the patient and can only be used for a short time.
9   When the wound has been thoroughly explored, remove any necrotic tissue or potentially necrotic tissue by excision with the scalpel. Trim ragged skin edges with the scalpel. Do not remove more tissue than is essential. When you are satisfied with your wound toilet, then suture and/or dress the wound as appropriate.

24

11 Wound toilet

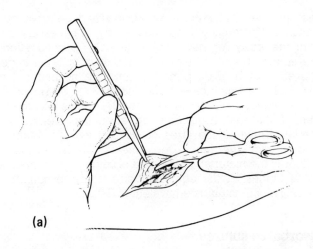

(a)

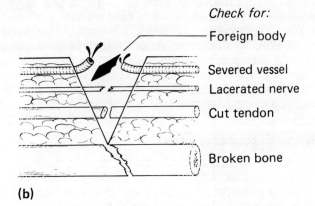

Check for:

Foreign body

Severed vessel
Lacerated nerve

Cut tendon

Broken bone

(b)

12 Suture materials

These are used for the closure of wounds and the repair of internal structures. They should not cause any unnecessary reactions within the body, or have any potentially harmful effects. The material may be non-absorbable, and such material is generally removed after a given period of time, or the material may be absorbable, in which case it does not have to be removed.

Suture materials come in various thicknesses and the different types of material have differing strengths. Generally, suture materials between the sizes of 6/0 and 2/0 are found in most Accident and Emergency Departments. The larger the number, the finer is the material. In the case of catgut, the number tends to be one higher for the equivalent size suture to non-absorbable sutures, i.e. 4/0 catgut is equivalent to 3/0 silk.

Absorbable sutures

Catgut

Catgut is manufactured from the sub-mucosal layer of sheep intestine, or the serosal layer of beef intestine.

Plain catgut loses half its strength in some 5–7 days and it has lost all its effective strength in about 12–18 days. Plain catgut tends to cause a considerable tissue reaction.

Chromic catgut loses half its strength within 17–21 days and it has lost all its effective strength by 28–32 days. It tends to cause less of a tissue reaction than plain catgut.

Synthetic absorbable sutures

There are various products on the market, such as polyglactin (Vicryl) and polyglycolic acid (Dexon). They have different handling properties compared with catgut, in that they tend to tie more easily, and they are slower to be absorbed.

Non-absorbable materials

Silk

This is probably the most commonly used material for skin closure. It comes as a braided material and it is easy to tie and work with.

12 Suture materials

Synthetic non-absorbable sutures

There are a variety of synthetic sutures which are non-absorbable. They may be monofilament materials such as polyamide (Ethilon) or polypropylene (Prolene) or they may be multi-filament materials. These sutures run through the tissues very easily, but the knots require extra ties as they tend to slip.

13 Suture needles

Surgical needles are made of stainless steel and there are now relatively few 'eyed' needles used. With eyed needles, they had to be threaded with the appropriate thread, and this would result in a greater bulk of needle and thread having to be pulled through the tissues at the level of the eye of the needle. They have therefore been replaced by 'atraumatic needles' in which the thread is already sealed into the end of the needle and these come as prepacked items with a given needle to a specific gauge and length of thread.

Needles can either be straight or come in a range of curves. The gauge of the needle will, to some extent, depend on the gauge of thread being used.

Round-bodied needles

These are needles with a round tapering tip. They are used to separate tissue fibres rather than to cut through tissues. They are used in soft tissues such as the intestine or in cardiovascular surgery.

Cutting needles

These have a cutting edge which allows them to pass easily through tough or dense tissues such as skin.

Trocar needles have a strong cutting edge, which merges into a round body. They are used for heavy work where the tissues tend to be tough.

Conventional cutting needle

These needles have a triangular cross section with the apex of the triangle on the inside of the needle curve. The cutting edges are restricted to the front section of the needle and they run into the triangular body of the needle which continues for half the length of the needle.

Reverse cutting needle

The body of this needle is triangular in cross section, but the apex of the cutting edge is on the outside of the needle curve. This makes the needle stronger, and helps the needle to resist bending.

13 Suture needles

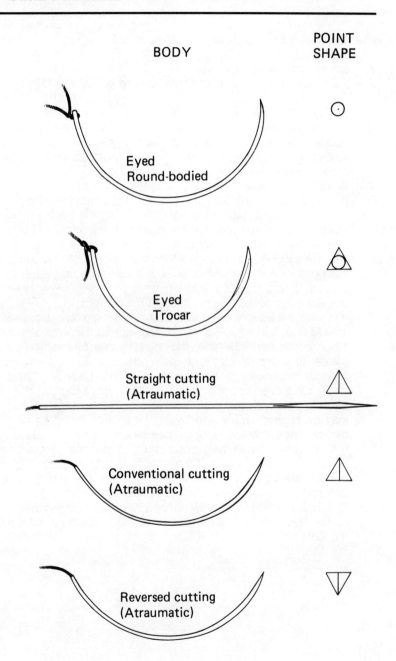

BODY

POINT
SHAPE

Eyed
Round-bodied

Eyed
Trocar

Straight cutting
(Atraumatic)

Conventional cutting
(Atraumatic)

Reversed cutting
(Atraumatic)

14 Principles of suturing

This describes the insertion of the sutures.

A   Suture pack (*see page 12*)
B   Suitable suture material and needle (*see pp. 26 and 28*)

1   The needle is held in the needle holder at a point approximately three-quarters of its length away from the needle tip (**a**). The needle itself is then at a right angle to the jaws of the needle holder. With the needle holder in the operators right hand the tip of the needle should be pointing to the left.
2   A curved needle should enter the skin so that its tip is perpendicular to the skin (**b**). This will result in the needle running to the required depth and its natural curvature will bring it into the wound as the operator gently supinates the hand holding the needle holder. It is the angle at which the needle enters the skin and the subsequent rotation which will determine the depth and the point of exit that the needle will take from the edge of the wound. Lifting the skin edge with forceps will help obtain the correct entry of the needle through the skin (**c**).
3   It is always a temptation to introduce the needle on one side of the wound and then try to run the needle across the wound so that it exits on the opposite side, thus making one bite suffice for the suture. In many cases, this is quite adequate, but if the wound is fairly large or deep, then the stitch will tend to be superficial, and it will leave a dead space below it. There is also a danger, that in an effort to pass the needle all the way across the wound, the needle may be pushed and levered so that it breaks. A further problem can be that if only the tip of the needle breaks through the skin on the opposite side of the wound and it is grasped by the needle holder, the cutting edge of the needle may be damaged. It is far wiser to take a large wound in two bites; one bite with the needle entering the skin on one side of the wound, and removing it at the bottom of the wound; and the second bite reintroducing the needle on the opposite side of the wound (**d**) and pushing it out through the skin (**e**).

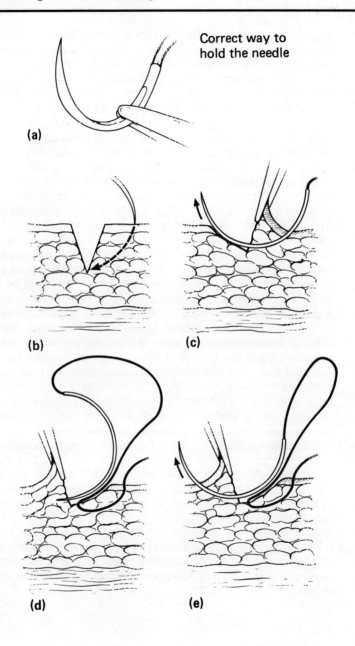

Correct way to
hold the needle

(a)

(b)

(c)

(d)

(e)

14 Principles of suturing

4   When a suture is made, the distance between the wound edge and the point of entry of the needle should be the same as between the wound edge and the exit point of the needle. The depth to which the needle has gone should be the same on both sides of the wound (**f**). When the stitch is made, the suture should be tied, either with the aid of forceps or with a surgeon's knot (**g**). The suture should not be too loose, nor should it be too tight. A tight suture will cause skin necrosis and this will be made worse by the fact that the wound tissues will swell after the suturing.

5   Individual sutures must be placed at even distances from each other, so that the wound is symmetrical in respect of the spacing of the sutures. As well as each of the sutures being symmetrical in its distance across the wound, all sutures should be of similar tension. The knots should be laid on one side of the wound.

6   In a situation where there is a deep wound, it may be impossible to close it in one layer. Where this is the case, a deep absorbable suture should be placed at regular intervals along deeper aspects of the wound, thus reducing the depth of the wound to be closed by the skin sutures. In such situations it is preferable to bury the knot, that is the stitch is put in 'upside down'. The reason for doing this is to put the knot as deep as possible because knots cause a greater tissue reaction. To carry this procedure out, the needle is introduced into the bottom of the wound with the needle exiting approximately half way up the edge of the wound (**h**), the needle is removed and then introduced at a similar level (half way) on the other side of the wound and pulled out at the bottom of the wound (**i**). This puts the ends of the suture at the bottom of the wound so the knot will be tied in the desired position (**j**).

7   In the case of a long wound, it is better to start with a central suture, which effectively divides the wound into two, and then possibly two further sutures, each placed half way between the middle suture and the opposite ends of the wound. This will enable further sutures to be placed at even intervals and will give the wound a neater appearance.

8   If there is some slight tension in a wound, one method of reducing it is to work from each end of the wound, placing alternate sutures at alternate ends. As the wound is closed towards its centre, the tension is reduced, so allowing neat approximation of the wound edges.

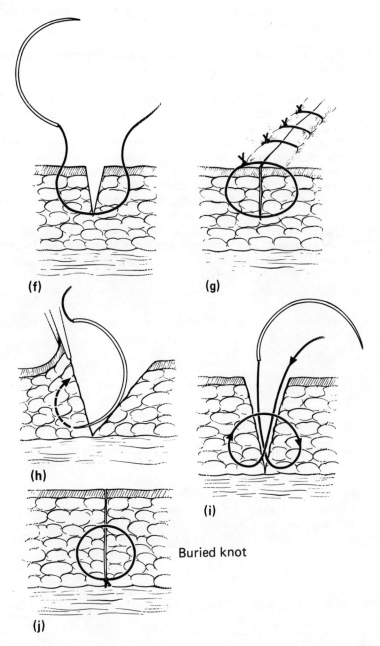

(f)

(g)

(h)

(i)

(j)

Buried knot

15 Instrument tying of sutures

This is the routine method for tying sutures with the aid of needleholders.

A   You will already have all the equipment required in the suture pack

1   After inserting the suture (**a**) and (**b**), the needleholders should be in the right hand. The end of the suture with the needle attached is held in the left hand.

2   Place the needleholders on top of the strand of the suture held in the left hand (**c**). Loop the suture material around the tip of the needleholders twice (**d**).

3   Pick up the free end of the suture with the needleholders (**e**). By slipping the loops off the end of the needleholders draw this end through the loops. This produces the first 'half hitch'.

4   Tighten down the 'half hitch' so that the wound edges are gently approximated. This involves crossing your hands, left in front of right (**f**).

15 Instrument tying of sutures

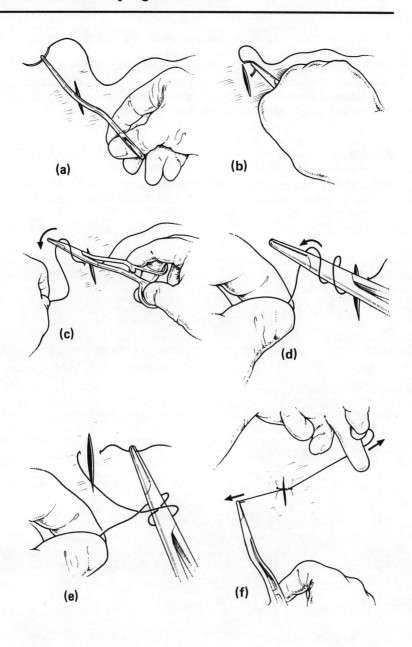

(a)

(b)

(c)

(d)

(e)

(f)

15 Instrument tying of sutures

5   Now uncross your hands and this rotates the 'half hitch' through 180 degrees and locks the 'half hitch' (**g**).

6   Let go of the end of the suture with the needleholders. Place the needleholders under the strand held in the left hand (**h**). Loop the suture material around the tip of the needleholders once (**i**). Then repeat as in 3 above to produce the second 'half hitch' (**j**).

7   Tighten the knot, but do not pull it so hard that the skin edges are crushed together (**k**).

8   If using a smooth suture material then put a further 'half hitch' on the knot to keep it tight.

9   Cut the suture ends to the required length (about 1 cm unless longer ends are required for a particular reason, i.e. in skin grafting).

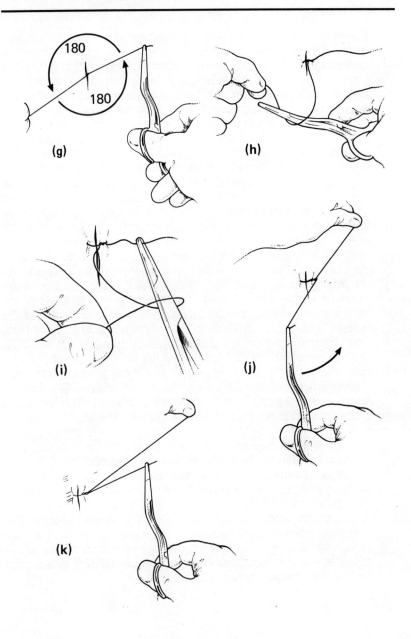

(g)

(h)

(i)

(j)

(k)

16 Problems in wound closure

There may be situations where there has been some skin loss. It may still be possible to close the wound if the wound edges are undermined. To do this, evert one side of the wound and with a scalpel blade, run the blade along the length of the wound, just below the dermis (**a**) and (**b**). Take care not to cut through the skin. If this cut is made too superficially, then the blood supply of the skin flap will be embarrassed. Repeat the manoeuvre on the opposite side of the wound and this should allow the wound edges to be approximated without tension.

When wound edges fail to sit in a neat fashion and there is a step, first try to eliminate the step by drawing the knot across to the opposite side of the wound, as this often tends to realign the wound and make it sit more neatly. If it is obvious that the skin edges are tending to curl inwards and that plain suturing is not going to be effective, then vertical mattress sutures should be used.

To perform a vertical mattress suture, a stitch is made as already described, but then the needle is reintroduced at the very edge of the wound on one side and then taken through and out of the opposite edge of the wound. This means that both ends of the suture material are now on one side of the wound (**c**). As the tension is placed on this suture, the wound edges are brought into neat approximation with a slight degree of eversion (**d**).

Flap wounds are a problem in that the tip of the flap will have a poor blood supply and it should not be directly sutured, as this will further embarrass the blood supply. In a 'V' shaped flap wound, each edge is sutured from the base towards the tip. The last suture is then placed in one side of the skin opposite the tip of the flap, the needle is drawn out of the wound edge and it is gently passed through the subcutaneous tissue of the tip of the flap, and then through the skin on the opposite side of the wound (**e**). When this suture is tightened to the necessary tension, the tip of the flap will be neatly approximated in the 'V', but there will be no tension on the tip of skin itself (**f**).

This principle can be applied to 'T' and 'Y' shaped wounds. The important point is that where there is a triangular tip to a flap, this should be sutured in a subcutaneous manner, and where two of these tips come together, each should be sutured in a similar fashion and the suture tied across healthy skin (**g**) and (**h**).

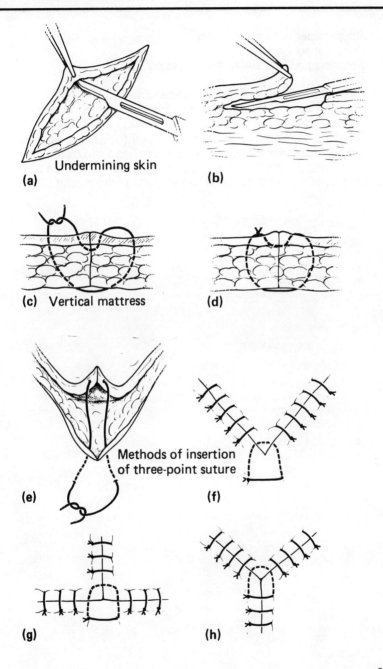

(a) Undermining skin

(b)

(c) Vertical mattress

(d)

(e)

Methods of insertion of three-point suture

(f)

(g)

(h)

17 Removing sutures

A   Suture scissors or stitch cutter
B   Non-toothed forceps
C   Dressing pack, or swabs and cleaning solution

1   Clean the wound and remove scabs and debris.
2   Hold the knot of the suture in the forceps. Cut the suture on the opposite side of the wound close to the skin (**a**).
3   Draw the 'knot' end of the suture across the wound to remove the suture. This prevents the wound being pulled apart by the removal of the suture. By cutting the suture close to the skin, only a minimal amount of 'external' suture is drawn through the wound.

17 Removing sutures

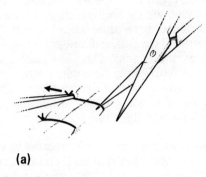

(a)

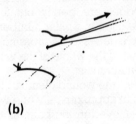

(b)

18 Skin closure: 'adherent strips'

There are various proprietary products on the market. These adherent strips come in varying widths and are about 5 cm long. There are several strips contained in the same sealed packet. The strips are used to close superficial wounds, remembering that they will not control any deep wound spaces. They are particularly valuable in children as they can obviously be applied without the distress and discomfort of a local anaesthetic, followed by suturing. They are not effective across the skin creases at joints due to movement of the joint which loosens the strip.

1   Clean and dry the edges of the wound carefully. Protect the wound itself with a piece of gauze and spray the skin on each side of the wound with tincture of benzoin, as this will give a sticky surface.
2   Open the sterile pack and remove one of the adherent tapes. Apply the tape to the centre of the wound so that half its length is stuck down on one side, and then with gentle tension, adhere the tape to the opposite side of the wound. Repeat this manoeuvre, but start the next tape on the opposite side of the wound and draw the tension in the opposite direction. Thus the tension is alternated along the wound, and the wound edges are gently but firmly approximated (a). The tapes should be used in similar numbers to sutures. There is no place for multiple tapes criss-crossing the wound, as this produces an untidy result. If the whole of the wound is covered by tapes, it will tend to remain moist.
3   The patient should be instructed to keep the wound clean and dry and not to remove the dry dressing until approximately one week has passed. The tapes can then be removed in the bath, as they will tend to float off. When the patient is removing the tapes, they must be warned to remove them by lifting each end of the tape and drawing them up simultaneously towards the centre of the wound (b). This will prevent any tension being placed across the wound and there will be no tendency to pull the wound open.

18 Skin closure: 'adherent strips'

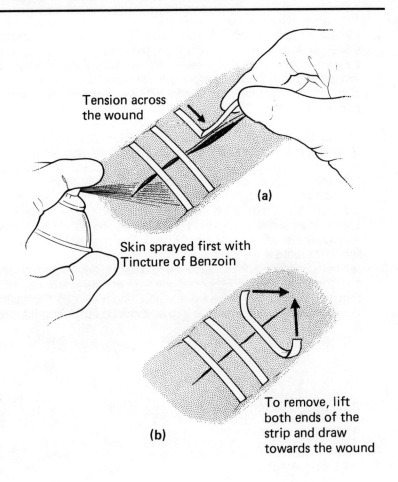

Tension across the wound

Skin sprayed first with Tincture of Benzoin

(a)

To remove, lift both ends of the strip and draw towards the wound

(b)

19 Skin closure: clips

Metal clips can be applied to a wound. They approximate the skin edges, and they do not tend to leave the 'cross hatching' that may be seen from suturing, so a neater scar results. There are various proprietary pre-packed disposable systems (**a**) and (**b**). They contain a set number of clips of a given size, which are inserted from a dispenser.

1   Michel clips are used in surgery. The clips are loaded onto a special forcep, which is used to approximate skin edges, and which is held in the operator's left hand. Application forceps are held in the right hand (**c**). The forceps in the right hand pick up a clip and place it across the wound (**d**) and then crimp the clip (**e**). The left hand moves down the wound using the forceps to approximate the skin edges, as further clips are placed across the wound by the forceps in the right hand. The spacing of the clips is similar to sutures.

2   Michel clips are left in place for 5–7 days, depending on the situation of the wound. Special forceps are required for their removal. The beak of these forceps goes under the clip. Closure of the forceps wedges opens the clip so it can be lifted from the skin (**f**).

19 Skin closure: clips

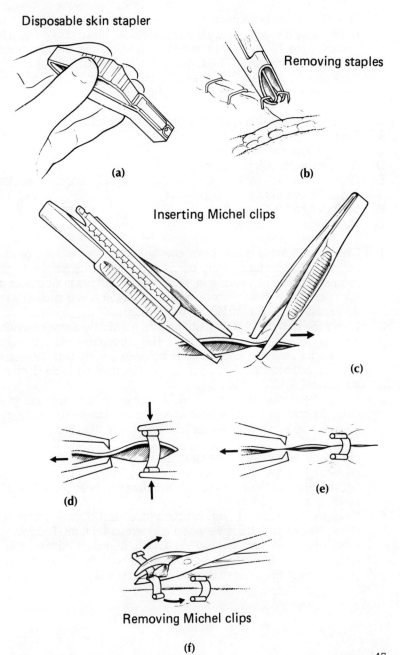

Disposable skin stapler

Removing staples

(a)

(b)

Inserting Michel clips

(c)

(d)

(e)

Removing Michel clips

(f)

20 Skin grafting

Split skin grafting enables an area of full thickness skin loss to be covered by a piece of partial thickness skin from a donor site. The grafted area heals in approximately 1 week and the donor site should heal over in. 10–14 days. As the donor site is partial thickness, it epithelializes over its total area and not just from the skin edges, as would happen in a full thickness skin defect.

A   A small Humby skin grafting knife, or Silva's knife
B   Two skin grafting boards
C   Three pieces of para-tulle
D   A suture pack. 4/0 suture material
E   20 ml of 0.5 per cent lignocaine with 1:200 000 adrenaline. Also some 0.5 per cent plain lignocaine
F   Syringes and 23G needles
G   Dressings and bandages

1   Choose a suitable donor site close to the area where the graft is needed. The texture of the donor skin should be similar to the recipient site. The donor site will not scar, but it will discolour so take account of the cosmetic effect. Common donor sites are the thigh and the flexor surface of the forearm.

2   Clean the skin of the donor site and then infiltrate a square of skin with the local anaesthetic solution. The adrenaline will blanch the skin so the anaesthetized area can be seen. Ensure that the area of skin anaesthetized is large enough so the grafting knife does not cut unanaesthetized skin (**a**).

3   Clean the donor site again with a solution which does not stain (e.g., Savlon) so the pale area of skin is not obscured. Towel the area, leaving an adequate surface free to cut the graft.

4   Grease the donor site with a piece of para-tulle and then grease the blade and roller of the grafting knife. Place another piece of para-tulle on one of the boards.

5   Set the roller of the knife, so that the distance between roller and blade is about 0.5 mm.

6   Take the other board (with no para-tulle) and draw it across the donor site so the skin is flattened and stretched tight. Follow with the knife about 2 cm behind the board, and start cutting with a gentle to-and-fro motion. Concentrate on the side to side movement of the knife and gently advance it (**b**).

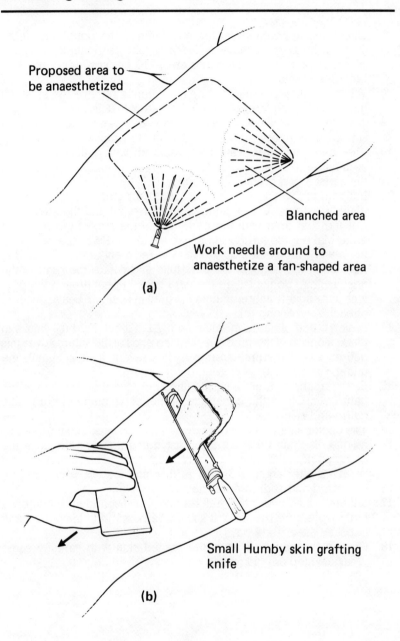

Proposed area to
be anaesthetized

Blanched area

Work needle around to
anaesthetize a fan-shaped area

(a)

Small Humby skin grafting
knife

(b)

7 Check the appearance of the cut skin and the donor site. If the graft is the correct thinness there should be multiple pin-point bleeding points over the donor area. Thicker grafts produce less bleeding points.

8 When a sufficient area has been cut, gently remove the knife, lift the cut skin with forceps and cut it free with scissors.

9 Lay this skin on the para-tulle on the board with the glistening cut surface uppermost. Smooth the skin out to its maximum extent.

10 The recipient area can be prepared with saline soaks for 30 minutes. This stops bleeding in a fresh wound, or helps clean the surface of a granulating wound.

11 Infiltrate the wound edges of the recipient area with 0.5 per cent plain lignocaine. Clean the area and towel around the area.

12 Cut the skin graft with the para-tulle to the size of the recipient area. Make it too large rather than too small. Place the graft with the freshly cut surface down onto the recipient area.

13 Peel back the edge of the para-tulle and suture the graft to the healthy skin. Do not suture the para-tulle. Repeat around the graft with just enough sutures to hold the graft in position. Leave one end of each suture long (c).

14 Soak a piece of gauze in saline and wring it out. Fold the gauze to place it on top of the graft. Tie the long ends of the sutures over this gauze. This 'pressure' dressing will prevent fluid accumulating under the graft (d).

15 Clean around the recipient site and apply a dry dressing over the gauze etc. Clean the donor site and apply a piece of para-tulle, gauze and bandage to it.

16 The doctor should remove his own dressings after about 5 days, so no-one else can be accused of dislodging the graft. Remove the gauze pack at this time, but leave the sutures. The sutures can be removed after another 3 days. At this time the donor site can be inspected and redressed as necessary.

17 If there is fluid under the graft remove it by aspiration, and apply a further pressure dressing. It should be possible to leave the graft exposed after 10–12 days.

18 Caution the patient to treat the grafted skin with care for some weeks to stop any damage.

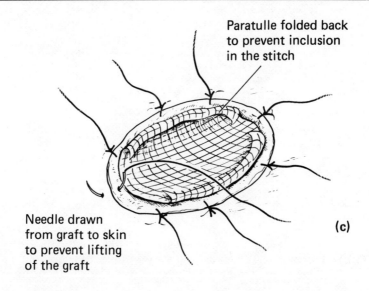

Paratulle folded back
to prevent inclusion
in the stitch

Needle drawn
from graft to skin
to prevent lifting
of the graft

(c)

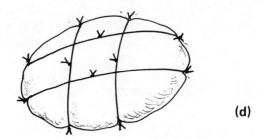

(d)

The long ends of the
sutures are tied over
the gauze swab

Section 2
Vascular access

21 Venepuncture

This is used to take venous blood samples, or it can be used to give intravenous injections.

A   Tourniquet
B   Syringe of appropriate size
C   Needle of 21G and 4 cm in length
D   Blood bottles as appropriate
E   Mediswab (skin cleanser)

1   Apply the tourniquet to the upper arm, making sure that it is not too tight. (The pressure should be less than the diastolic blood pressure).
2   Select a vein which is prominent on the upper limb. Generally the antecubital fossa is the most satisfactory site.
3   If the veins are not obvious, tap the skin which overlies the antecubital fossa and this may help dilate the veins. If there are no suitable veins, try the other arm.
4   Take the syringe and free the plunger by moving it up and down the syringe barrel. Attach the needle with the bevel facing upwards.
5   Clean the skin in the area of the vein
6   Approach the vein with the needle directed along the vein at an angle of some 10–15 degrees to the skin (*see illustration*). Pass the needle through the skin and into the vein. The needle should pass approximately a centimetre along the inside of the vein after insertion. Draw back gently on the syringe plunger and take the appropriate volume of blood.
7   Remove the tourniquet from the upper arm and apply gentle pressure with a Mediswab over the puncture site and withdraw the needle. Continue to apply pressure and apply a plaster as necessary.
8   Causes of failure may be
    (a) The needle has missed the vein. If this has happened withdraw the needle and start again.
    (b) The needle has passed right through the vein. If this has happened slowly withdraw the needle whilst applying gentle traction to the syringe plunger. When the needle re-enters the vein blood can be withdrawn and the needle can be gently passed further along the vein.

Complications

If the vein has been 'nicked' by the needle a haematoma quickly forms around the vein. It is best to apply pressure to this site, remove the tourniquet and needle and try another vein.

21 Venepuncture

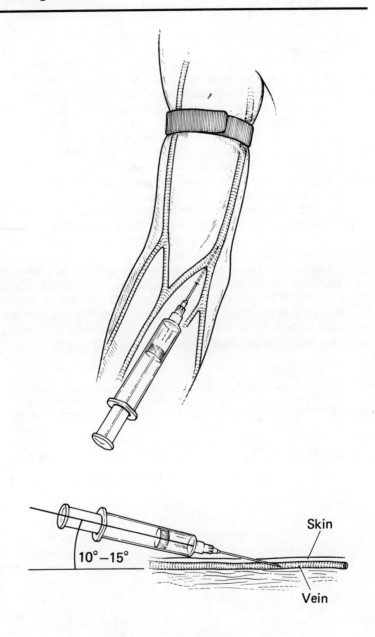

Skin

10°–15°

Vein

22 Intravenous fluids

These come in various forms of containers. The commonest is a plastic bag (**a**), which is contained within an outer plastic bag that must first be removed. The bag of the IV fluid will have a port for the giving set connector, which will usually have some sort of seal on it which must be penetrated by the sharp plastic spike of the giving set. There is generally a further port with a rubber end on it, through which drugs etc. can be injected into the intravenous fluid. The bag can be hung directly onto a drip stand. There can be various modifications of these principles and a careful inspection of the bag before starting is advised.

More rigid plastic containers such as 'polyfusers' (**b**) have become more common. To connect these to the giving set, the top is snapped off and the bottle must be sitting top uppermost when this is done, as there is no further valve mechanism. The plastic spike of the giving set is gently pushed into the open end of the polyfuser bottle.

Haemaccel (**c**), which is commonly used in situations where there has been blood loss, has a different mechanism. There is a ring on top of the plastic bottle which must be pulled off and this reveals a hole under which a rubber diaphragm is situated. The plastic spike of the giving set is pushed through the opening and then has to penetrate the rubber diaphragm.

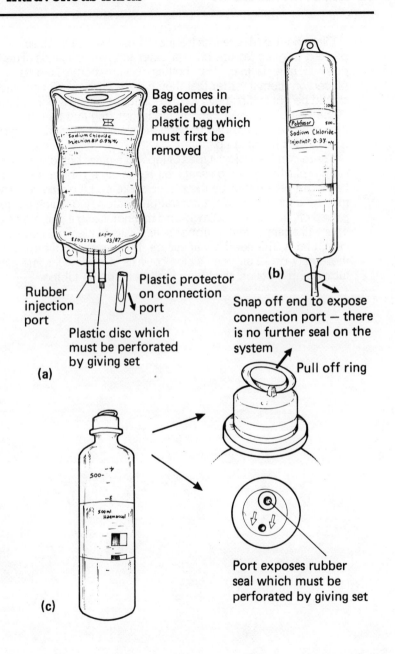

Bag comes in a sealed outer plastic bag which must first be removed

Rubber injection port

Plastic protector on connection port

Plastic disc which must be perforated by giving set

(a)

(b)

Snap off end to expose connection port — there is no further seal on the system

Pull off ring

(c)

Port exposes rubber seal which must be perforated by giving set

Glass bottles (**d**) are less frequently used now, but plasma is still packed in glass, as are certain other intravenous fluids. The first point to note is that glass bottles require bottle holders to be placed on them in order that they can be hung up. These holders should be put on first before connecting the giving set. The bottom of the bottle is passed through the larger ring and then the top of the bottle can be slipped through the smaller ring and the system is ready for hanging up.

There can be various types of tops on a glass bottle. It may be a simple plastic top which snaps off revealing a rubber seal, which has to be penetrated by the plastic spike of the giving set. There may be a metal top with a central perforated ring which has to be prised off, in a somewhat awkward manner, using a pair of scissors. This will again reveal a rubber seal. Glass bottles will need an air vent, and a 21G needle will suffice. However with the giving set there may be an air vent, which consists of a needle, some plastic tubing and a cotton wool plug in the end of the tubing.

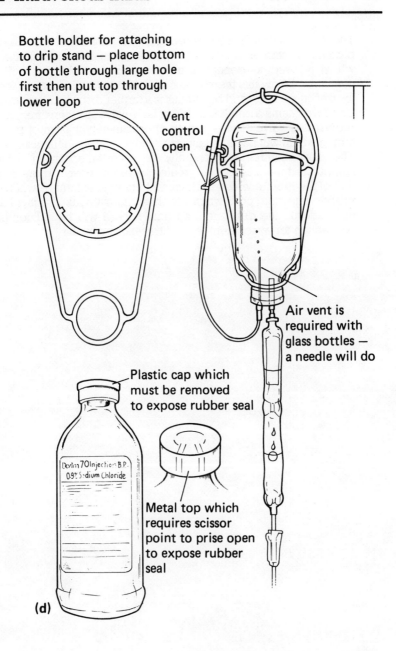

Bottle holder for attaching to drip stand — place bottom of bottle through large hole first then put top through lower loop

Vent control open

Air vent is required with glass bottles — a needle will do

Plastic cap which must be removed to expose rubber seal

Devlin 70 Injection B.P. 0.9% Sodium Chloride

Metal top which requires scissor point to prise open to expose rubber seal

(d)

23 Giving sets

There are various designs of giving set on the market, but they all basically consist of some form of plastic spike at the proximal end which is used to penetrate any seal on the IV infusion fluid container. Below this there is a drip chamber which contains some form of gauze filter, and below this is a further drip chamber, which usually contains a small ball to act as a valve, or there may be a rubber flap valve. There is then approximately 150 cm of plastic tubing which will have an adjustable flow control mechanism on it. The flow control is generally a roller mechanism which compresses the tubing to a greater or lesser extent. At the distal end of the tubing, which is attached to the patient, there will be a rubber injection port which enables intravenous drugs to be injected into the drip line, and finally there will be a Luer Lok connection for attachment to an intravenous cannula.

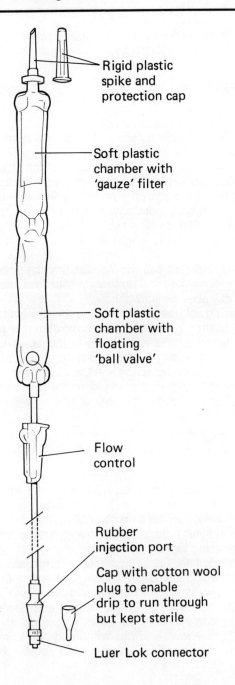

Rigid plastic
spike and
protection cap

Soft plastic
chamber with
'gauze' filter

Soft plastic
chamber with
floating
'ball valve'

Flow
control

Rubber
injection port

Cap with cotton wool
plug to enable
drip to run through
but kept sterile

Luer Lok connector

24 Setting up a drip

This is a basic principle for 'running a drip through' in preparation for giving an infusion to a patient through an intravenous cannula.

A   A giving set (*see page 58*)
B   Intravenous fluid (*see page 54*)
C   A drip stand

1   Select the fluid that you are going to infuse, check that it is correct and that it is in date. Take the giving set and remove it from its cellophane wrapper.
2   Remove the plastic cover from the sharp plastic spike of the giving set and remove any plastic covering from the port on the IV fluid bag. Holding the bag with the ports uppermost, gently drive the plastic spike down the connector port, until it perforates the seal and enters the bag. Check that the flow control is fully occluding the tubing before turning the bag upside-down and hanging it on the drip stand.
3   Squeeze the bag gently and fluid will run through first the upper and then the lower drip chambers and do this until approximately half of the lower drip chamber contains fluid.
4   Raise the end of the giving set (the patient end) to the level of the bag and open the flow control. This allows fluid to run along the full length of the plastic tubing until it just comes to the tip of the connector. If this is done carefully, it avoids wasting fluid and it eliminates any air bubbles from the giving set. Carefully hang the end of the giving set, with its cover in place, over the drip stand where it will be ready for attaching to the patient when a cannula has been placed in a vein.
5   Then proceed to Venous cannulation (*see page 62*).

Complications

If air bubbles appear in the tubing, they can either be removed by running fluid through the system, but this is wasteful, or the bubbles can be tapped back into the drip chamber. The latter is best done by holding the plastic tubing straight in a vertical fashion and tapping it with something like a pair of scissors.

If the lower chamber becomes full of fluid, then it is impossible to determine the rate at which the drip is running. To empty this chamber, remove the bag from the drip stand and hold it upside-down and then squeeze both the upper and lower chambers until they are empty. Allow the chambers to expand, whilst the bag is still upside-down and this will empty the lower chamber. It can then be correctly filled as described above.

24 Setting up a drip

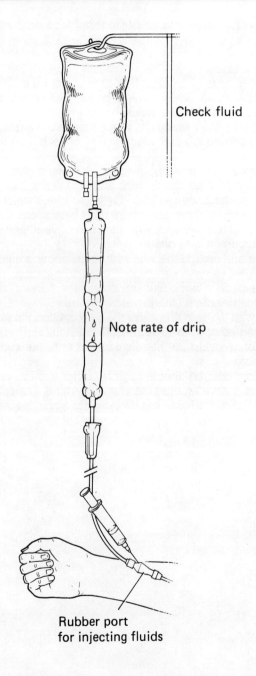

Check fluid

Note rate of drip

Rubber port
for injecting fluids

25 Venous cannulation

This is used to provide routine infusion of fluids or blood products.

A   Tourniquet
B   Skin preparation materials
C   A protective sheet (plastic or an inconti-pad) to protect the bed
D   Appropriate sized cannulas, always have a spare. 18G for routine use, but 16G or preferably 14G for resuscitation.
E   An appropriate infusion fluid which has been attached to a giving set, that has been run through and which is free of air bubbles.

1   Apply the tourniquet to the upper arm. If the patient is right-handed endeavour to use the left arm, and *vice versa*. If there is an injured limb, use the uninjured limb. Try to use a vein which is as distal as possible on the limb and avoid veins over joints.
2   Cover the bedding under the arm with the protective sheeting. Tap the vein to encourage it to dilate.
3   Clean the skin over and around the vein with an antiseptic solution or a medi-wipe.
4   Open the cannula pack. Check that the cannula is fully on the needle, and turn the needle so the bevel is upwards.
5   Align the cannula with the vein and enter the vein through the skin with the cannula angled at 10 to 15 degrees to the skin (**a**). Do this in a positive fashion, moving the needle forward until the blood passes up the needle.
6   It is important to advance the needle slightly further into the vein as the point alone may have entered the vein at this time. Then slip the cannula off the needle (**b**) until its total length is within the vein (**c**).

25 Venous cannulation

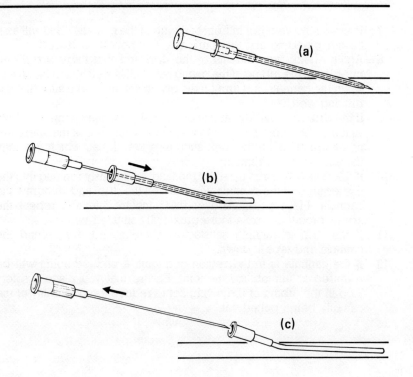

(a)

(b)

(c)

7 Press on the vein just in front of the tip of the cannula. This will stop further bleeding and the tourniquet can now be released.

8 Again check the contents of the drip and that there are no air bubbles in the tubing of the giving set. If all is well attach the giving set to the cannula and turn on the giving set and make sure that it is running well.

9 If the drip does not run at this point, withdraw the cannula slightly, as it may be impinging on the wall of the vein. Check that there are no obstructions on the limb such as a tourniquet, which you may have forgotten to remove.

10 If the drip fails to run freely or the fluid is obviously running into the tissues around the cannula, then turn off the drip, and withdraw the cannula. Place pressure over the puncture site and repeat the above procedure on a more proximally situated vein.

11 If the drip is running satisfactorily, clean and dry around the cannula and tape it down.

12 If the cannula is in the region of a joint, a padded splint will be required to immobilize the joint. Ensure that you place a safety loop in the tubing of the giving set to reduce the possibility of the cannula being pulled out.

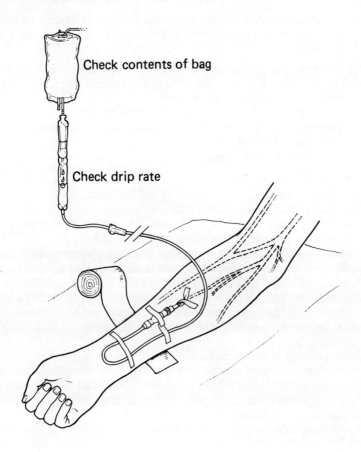

Check contents of bag

Check drip rate

26 Venous cut-down

This provides rapid access to a vein in an emergency situation where other 'puncture' techniques have failed or proved impossible.

A A cut-down pack: scalpel, scissors with sharp points, fine toothed forceps, plain forceps, two curved mosquito artery forceps, aneurysm needle and needle holder
B Plain 3/0 catgut. 3/0 silk on curved cutting needle
C Intravenous cannula: 18G to 12G depending on purpose
D Skin preparation and towels
E Syringe and normal saline

1 Locate the vein:
   (a) Long saphenous anterior to medial malleolus
   (b) Basilic in the antecubital fossa
2 Clean and towel the area. The vein may not be obvious so it is essential to be sure of the anatomical landmarks.
3 Make a transverse incision through the skin, approximately 3 cm long, over where the vein is thought to lie. Spread the wound with mosquito forceps and identify the vein.
4 Mobilize the vein by running the mosquito forceps (**a**) under it and place two catgut ties under the vein, clipping each tie. These can then be used to elevate the vein and the distal tie will control bleeding from the vein.
5 With pointed scissors, make a nick in the side of the vein (**b**).
6 Place the aneurysm needle into the nick and elevate gently (**c**). This opens the nick in the vein and the cannula can be pushed into the vein in the proximal direction. The cannula should be passed almost to its full length.
7 Gently aspirate or inject normal saline down the cannula to ensure that it is in the right situation.
8 Tie the cannula in with the proximal tie of catgut and tie the vein off distally with the distal tie.
9 Attach the intravenous giving set after rechecking the IV fluid and ensuring that it runs. If the drip fails to run, check
   (a) All connections.
   (b) The tip of the cannula is not against the wall of the vein – pull it back slightly.
   (c) There is no clot in the cannula – flush the cannula with a small volume of saline.
10 Tie in the cannula and approximate the wound edges with skin sutures.
11 Dress the wound and tape down the cannula and the distal part of the giving set.

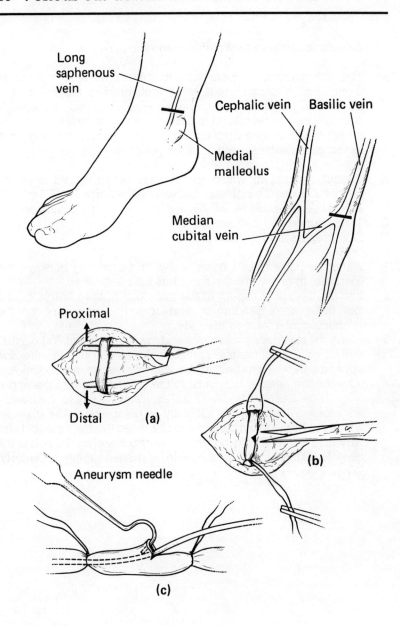

Long saphenous vein

Cephalic vein   Basilic vein

Medial malleolus

Median cubital vein

Proximal

Distal   (a)

(b)

Aneurysm needle

(c)

27 Central venous cannulation

Infraclavicular approach (subclavian vein)

This gives access to a central vein for central venous pressure monitoring. It allows drugs to be delivered to the heart. It is suitable for long-term parenteral feeding. It is a route by which a pacing wire can be placed in the right ventricle. The infraclavicular approach is more comfortable for the patient in the long-term, as the cannulation site is not in the neck.

A   Cannula system in which the cannula is introduced over the needle. Choose the right size cannula for the purpose (18G to 12G)
B   A No. 11 scalpel blade. 2/0 black silk on a straight cutting needle
C   10 ml syringe and 21G needle
D   Skin preparation materials and gloves

1   Place the patient head down and with a sand-bag between the scapulae, in order that the shoulders fall backwards.
2   Identify the lower aspect of the mid-point of the clavicle on the side that you are standing at. Next locate the upper aspect of the sternoclavicular joint on that side.
3   Clean the skin over a wide area and towel the patient. Take a 21G needle on a 10 ml syringe and push the needle through the skin approximately 1 cm below the clavicle at its mid-point and advance the needle, horizontal to the ground, towards the upper edge of the sterno-clavicular joint, aspirating gently as the needle advances. There may be difficulty in going under the clavicle, which is why the sandbag is placed between the scapulae and also why the needle should be placed approximately 1 cm below the clavicle, as this allows the needle to be pushed slightly posteriorly. When blood is aspirated freely withdraw the needle.

27 Central venous cannulation

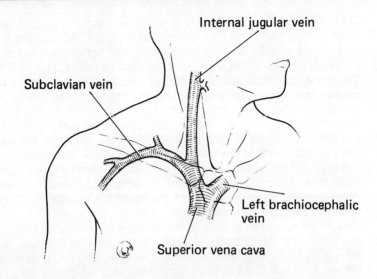

27 Central venous cannulation

4 Take the needle and its cannula with the syringe attached and advance it in the same line as that taken by the 21G needle. If a larger bore cannula is being used, it is as well to make a small nick in the skin, so as not to damage the leading edge of the cannula. The larger cannulas tend to push the vein slightly away and so a greater depth may be required before the vein is entered. On entering the vein and when there is a free aspiration of blood, advance the cannula and needle a few millimetres more, to ensure that the bevel of the needle is totally within the vein and then slip the cannula over the needle to its full length. Take the intravenous catheter and slip it down the cannula to its full depth. If there is any resistance to its progress, rotate the catheter gently. Many of these systems have some type of lock between the catheter and the cannula to ensure they stay connected.

5 Check the intravenous fluid, and that there is no air in the giving set, attach it to the catheter, still holding the catheter in place, and ensure that the drip is running, then lower the fluid bag below the patient to check that blood siphons freely into the giving set.

6 Clean around the puncture site and place a stitch through the skin and tie it to the cannula to ensure the cannula is not pulled out. Tape down the cannula and the distal part of the giving set.

7 Return the patient to the horizontal level and take an early chest X-ray to exclude any pneumothorax and to determine the exact position of the catheter.

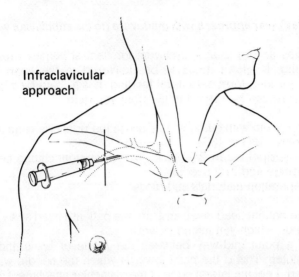

Infraclavicular
approach

28 Central venous cannulation

Supraclavicular approach with guidewire (to the subclavian vein)

This gives access to a central vein for central venous pressure monitoring. It allows drugs to be delivered to the heart. It is suitable for long-term parenteral feeding. It is a route by which a pacing wire can be placed in the right ventricle.

A Cannula system with guide wire. Choose the right size cannula for the purpose (18G to 12G)
B A No. 11 scalpel blade. 2/0 black silk on a straight cutting needle
C 10 ml syringe and 21G needle
D Skin preparation materials and gloves

1 Place the patient head down and turn the patient's head away from the side on which you intend to work.
2 Identify a point mid-way between the Angle of Louis and the sternal notch. This is the point towards which the needle will be advanced. Feel the lateral edge of the clavicular attachment of the sterno-mastoid muscle, by placing a finger between it and the posterior aspect of the clavicle. The needle puncture is made in this angle, approximately 1 cm behind the clavicle.
3 Clean the skin over a wide area, so enabling you to check all the landmarks as you progress. Take a 21G needle on a 10 ml syringe and positioning it as described above, push the needle in a horizontal fashion towards the mid-point of the manubrium. Aspirate gently as the needle goes in, until such time as a steady flow of blood is obtained. If the needle fails to locate the vein then try advancing it in the same line but 5 degrees anteriorly or posteriorly.
4 Take the needle from the cannulation set and place it on a 10 ml syringe. Remove the 21G needle and advance the cannulation needle in the same direction as this needle followed. It will tend to have to go a little deeper, as the larger needle pushes the wall of the vein away. Take care not to push the needle through into the chest. Aspirate gently as the needle is advanced, until a flow of blood is achieved, then pass the needle into the vein a little further to ensure that the bevel of the needle is completely through the wall of the vein.

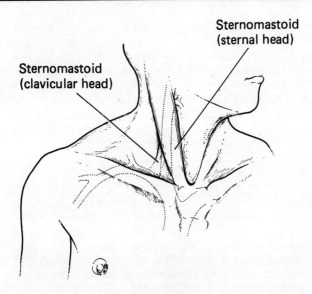

Sternomastoid
(sternal head)

Sternomastoid
(clavicular head)

28 Central venous cannulation

5   Check which end of the guide-wire is the 'soft' tip and run the guide wire down the inside of the needle. If it does not pass easily, rotate it gently, and if this fails then withdraw the guide-wire and aspirate the needle to see if it is still within the vein. If there is still marked resistance abandon the attempt. If a large bore cannula is going to be used and the guide-wire has passed freely into the vein, then make a small nick in the skin where the guide-wire passes through, as this will make the passage of the cannula easier and will prevent damage to its leading edge.

6   Withdraw the needle over the guide-wire, making sure that there is sufficient guide-wire outside the skin to allow the full length of the cannula to be fed over it and permitting the end of the guide-wire to be held as the cannula is fed down into the vein.

7   When the cannula is in place, remove the guide-wire and hold the cannula in place. Check the IV fluid, ensure that there are no bubbles in the giving set, and then connect it to the cannula. Ensure that there is a free flow of fluid, then lower the IV fluid bottle or bag below the patient and make sure that there is a free back-flow of blood into the giving set, thus ensuring that the cannula is resting in a vein. Run the drip at the required rate.

8   Clean around the puncture site and place a stitch through the skin and tie it to the cannula to ensure the cannula is not pulled out. Tape down the cannula and the distal part of the giving set.

9   Return the patient to the horizontal level and take an early chest X-ray to exclude any pneumothorax and to determine the exact position of the cannula.

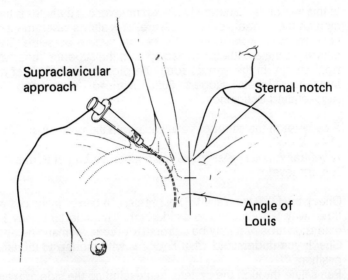

Supraclavicular approach

Sternal notch

Angle of Louis

29 Central venous pressure monitoring

In this technique, a centrally placed intravenous catheter is used to monitor the central venous pressure. This allows assessment of the need for fluid replacement. The central venous pressure (CVP) is measured via a catheter whose tip is in the superior vena cava or right atrium. In the normal adult, the pressure is 6–8 cm of water. Increasing levels suggest fluid overload, decreasing levels suggest fluid deficiency.

A A catheter in the superior vena cava, with the position checked on chest X-ray
B A central venous pressure monitor set and a bag of normal saline
C A spirit level

1 Check the CVP set. All CVP sets conist of a basic 'giving set' with a three-way tap attached to a side limb. The side limb may be an extension tube or it may be a properly graduated manometer tube. Check you understand what happens with the tap in its different positions.
2 Run saline through the system, first excluding the side arm and so filling the system like a giving set. When all air is excluded, turn the tap to connect the side arm to the saline and half fill the side arm. Some sets have a cotton wool plug as a filter at the top of the side arm. If the cotton wool becomes wet the saline in the side arm will not level properly when the CVP is measured.
3 Turn the tap to connect the patient limb to the saline bag, and connect the system to the IV catheter in the patient, having checked yet again that there is no air in the tube and there is normal saline in the bag.
4 Place the patient flat in the bed and mark a point in the mid-axillary line, this will remain the zero point for all CVP readings on the patient.
5 The side limb of the CVP set is placed in a vertical position up the drip stand and held by tape. Its lower aspect should be some 10 cm below the patient's mid-axillary line.

29 Central venous pressure monitoring

Tap position

1. Fill manometer tube

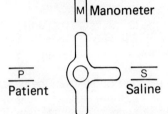

2. Connect manometer to patient

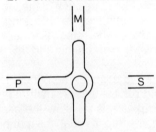

3. Run as a drip

6   With the spirit level, mark the horizontal level between the patient's zero point in the mid-axillary line and the manometer. Put a piece of tape on the manometer at this level and clearly mark it as zero.

7   Turn the CVP set's tap to connect the saline to the manometer and fill the manometer to about 20 cm above zero.

8   Turn the tap to connect the patient to the manometer and allow the manometer level to drop.

9   The level will oscillate due to changes in pressure in the superior vena cava, resulting from respiration and the cardiac cycle. If the level fails to oscillate, the IV catheter is not in a central vein. If the oscillations are very vigorous, the catheter may be in the right ventricle. If the level fails to drop, check the position of the tap and its various connections. Check if anything is blocking the manometer tube, such as a wet cotton wool plug. Normally the level will slowly drop to a point between 6 and 10 cm and this is the CVP reading.

10 After taking the reading, turn the tap to connect the patient to the saline, as for a normal giving set and run the saline slowly. Try and make 500 ml last 12 hours. If the drip rate is too slow the cannula will block, and if you fail to turn the tap so that the patient is disconnected from the manometer limb, then again the cannula will block. Do not leave the tap in a position whereby all the limbs are in communication, as this does not give an accurate CVP reading.

11 Each time the reading is repeated, the patient must be laid flat in the same position and the zero point checked on the manometer tube by using the spirit level.

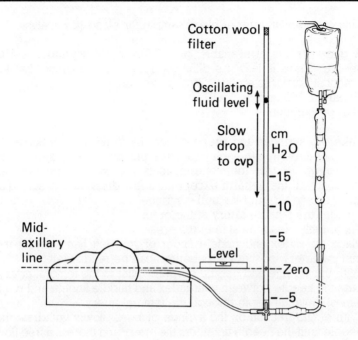

Cotton wool filter

Oscillating fluid level

Slow drop to cvp

cm H_2O

−15

−10

−5

Mid-axillary line

Level

−−Zero

−−5

30 Arterial puncture

This provides an arterial blood sample for blood gas analysis.

A A glass syringe, if available, or a 2.5 ml plastic syringe. A 21G needle. There is less gas diffusion from a glass syringe, but for practical purposes a plastic syringe will do.

B Heparin (5000 units in 1 ml)

C Skin preparation

1 Take two syringes and prepare them by drawing approximately 0.5 ml of heparin into each. Move the plunger of each syringe up and down so that the heparin coats the wall of the syringe. Eliminate all the heparin except for a few drops and ensure that there are no air bubbles in the syringe.

2 Feel for the femoral artery at the groin.

3 Thoroughly clean the skin in the area.

4 Place the index and middle finger of your left hand across the femoral artery, so that the pulsations can be readily felt.

5 With the syringe and needle perpendicular to the femoral artery, pass the needle between your index and middle fingers and run it almost to its full depth through the femoral artery.

6 With gentle traction on the syringe plunger, slowly withdraw the needle until the needle tip enters the artery and there is a free flow of blood into the syringe. Depending on the state of oxygenation of the patient, this blood is usually bright red and readily identified as arterial blood. In resuscitation situations where the pulse may have been difficult to feel and oxygenation is poor, then it may not be so easy to identify the blood as arterial.

7 If the blood that has been taken is of doubtful origin, remove the needle from the syringe, but leave the needle within the artery. Cap the syringe with a fresh needle to reduce the exposure of the blood to air. Look at the hub of the needle that is within the artery. If the needle is in the artery, there will be pulsation at the drop of blood which has formed in the hub of the needle. A fresh heparinized syringe should be attached to the needle and a further sample of blood taken. Be careful not to draw any air into the syringe.

8 Withdraw the needle and apply pressure over the puncture site, for approximately five minutes. Make sure the blood sample is analyzed immediately. If the sample has to go to a laboratory, place a cap over the end of the syringe, or bend the syringe needle to occlude its lumen. Pack the syringe in ice.

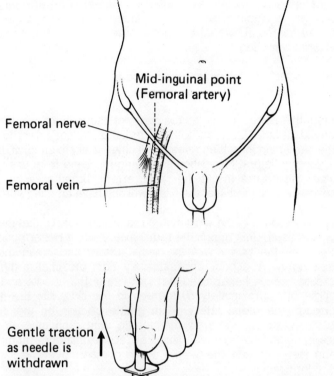

Mid-inguinal point
(Femoral artery)

Femoral nerve

Femoral vein

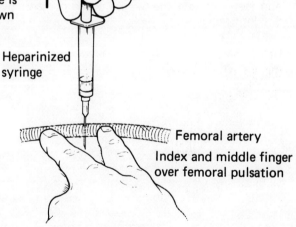

Gentle traction
as needle is
withdrawn

Heparinized
syringe

Femoral artery

Index and middle finger
over femoral pulsation

31 Radial artery stab

This is an alternative technique for obtaining an arterial blood sample. A cannula can also be placed at this site in the radial artery for radial arterial blood pressure monitoring or continuous arterial sampling.

A See under arterial puncture (*see page 80*). Prepare the syringe with heparin as described

1 Find the radial artery at the wrist of the patient, on his least dominant side. Occlude both the radial and ulnar artery to see if the hand blanches, then release the ulnar artery to check if there is a good collateral circulation supplying the hand from this vessel. This will ensure that if the radial artery thromboses, or if it is severely damaged, that the hand will still have an adequate blood supply.

2 Place the back of the wrist over a roll of bandage, so that the wrist is extended. This brings the radial artery into a better position.

3 Recheck the position of the radial artery and clean the skin thoroughly. At a point approximately 2 cm proximal to the wrist crease, take a heparinized syringe with a 21G needle and at an angle of approximately 60 degrees to the skin, run the needle through the radial artery. With gentle traction on the syringe plunger, slowly withdraw the needle until such time as blood freely enters the syringe. Withdraw approximately 2 ml of blood and then withdraw the needle. Place pressure over the puncture site for 5 minutes.

31 Radial artery stab

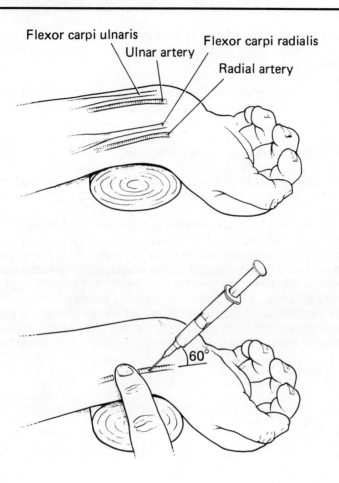

Flexor carpi ulnaris

Flexor carpi radialis

Ulnar artery

Radial artery

60°

32 Arterial blood pressure monitoring

A   A 20G cannula and needle to an arterial pressure 'kit'
B   500 ml of normal saline with 1000 units of heparin added, within a pressure bag.

1   Set up the arterial pressure kit in accordance with the instructions for the particular unit being used. These will include valves with a port for sampling, as well as a connection for attachment to a pressure transducer. The pressure in the bag of saline is kept above arterial systolic pressure (300 mm Hg).

2   Follow the procedures as laid out for radial artery stab (page 82), except that the needle and cannula should enter the skin at about 30 degrees to the skin. Impale the artery with the needle and cannula.

3   Very gently withdraw the needle and cannula, until there is a flash-back into the catheter. Now withdraw the needle and cannula a tiny bit more, to ensure that the bevel of the needle is within the artery and advance the cannula off the needle along the lumen of the artery. Withdraw the needle out of the cannula and apply pressure proximal to the cannula to control bleeding.

4   Attach the cannula to the pressure line, as set up, and apply the necessary dressings to immobilize the cannula and prevent it from being pulled out.

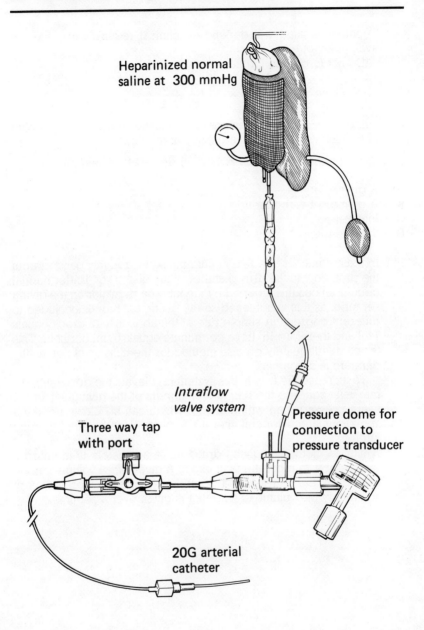

Heparinized normal
saline at 300 mmHg

*Intraflow
valve system*

Three way tap
with port

Pressure dome for
connection to
pressure transducer

20G arterial
catheter

33 Rate and volume control of infusions

Techniques used will depend on clinical requirements and the availability of equipment.

Do not forget the formula:

$$\text{Flow} = (Pa - Pb) \times \frac{\pi}{8} \times \frac{r^4}{zl}$$

where Pa − Pb is the pressure head, r is the radius and l the length of the cannula and z is the density of the fluid.

20 drops distilled water = 1 ml. 15 drops blood = 1 ml.

A A giving set
B A giving set with burette
C Infusion pump
D Syringe pump

1 In most situations, the rate of fluid infused is roughly gauged from the drop flow in the drip chamber of the giving set. Under normal circumstances this is varied by the infusion regulator on the giving set tube, as this is tightened so the giving set tube is occluded to different degrees. A simple rule of thumb is that 15 drops equals 1 ml and therefore 15 drops per minute equals 60 ml per hour. This is not an adequately precise method for the infusion of potentially dangerous drugs.

To increase the flow in this system (a) elevate the drip stand, (b) manually squeeze the bag and chambers of the giving set, or (c) use a pressure bag with a gauge, which can be blown up like a sphygmomanometer cuff after it has been placed around the bag of fluid.

2 A simple method of giving drugs more accurately is to utilize a giving set with a burette built into it. A given small volume can be placed in the burette and so it is possible to observe very accurately the volume of fluid that is given over a set time.

33 Rate and volume control of infusions

Burette system

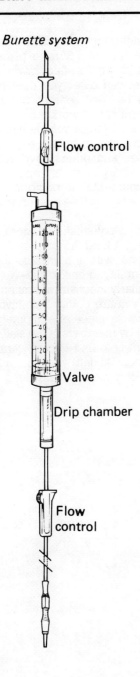

Flow control

Valve

Drip chamber

Flow
control

33 Rate and volume control of infusions

3 Syringe pumps are very accurate systems for giving small volumes of a fluid containing a drug. A syringe, usually of 20 ml, is placed in the apparatus and the plunger is slowly pushed down at a predetermined rate. As each system can differ you must make sure that you read the instructions or have somebody who is familiar with the apparatus to show you how it works.

4 Infusion pumps are useful for longer term, larger volume infusions. They all differ and each has its own requirements, e.g., some require a specific type of giving set, and others have volume chambers built in to the giving sets. They may only monitor the drop rate using a light sensor, and with a built in pump they can vary this rate. The more accurate types will infuse a given volume in a given time.

5 With the use of all solutions containing potentially dangerous or very potent drugs ensure that you have added the correct dosage to the correct volume in accordance with the manufacturer's instructions. It is the doctor's responsibility to check this.

6 With any piece of equipment, particularly mechanical equipment, ensure that you know exactly what you are doing. This involves reading the instructions for that particular piece of equipment, or being given specific instructions on it by members of the staff who are familiar with it. Equally important is to find out the common problems which cause that equipment to fail. Remember that neither verbal nor physical abuse rectify mechanical failure.

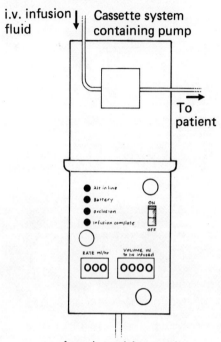

Infusion pump

i.v. infusion fluid

Cassette system containing pump

To patient

Air in line
Battery
occlusion
infusion complete

ON
OFF

RATE ml/hr

000

VOLUME ml to be infused

0000

Attach to drip stand

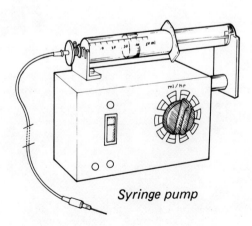

ml/hr

Syringe pump

Section 3
Airway procedures

34 Maintaining an airway

This is a basic technique which is used in the unconscious patient who is unable to maintain their own airway.

A No special equipment is required, but if available a Guedel Airway of suitable size is used (size 3 = adult female, size 4 = adult male)

1 Open the patient's mouth, remove dentures and any foreign material that is in the mouth or at the back of the throat.
2 Tilt the head backwards. Pull the lower jaw upwards, this draws the tongue forwards from the pharynx.
3 If it is available, insert a Guedel Airway (**a**) of appropriate size. This will help to keep the tongue forwards, off the back of the pharynx. Open the mouth and insert the airway over the tongue with 180 degrees rotation (**b**). If oxygen is available, hold the angles of the jaw forwards, and apply a face mask with an approximate gas flow of 10 ℓ per minute.
4 Ensure that the patient is making a respiratory effort by observing the chest.

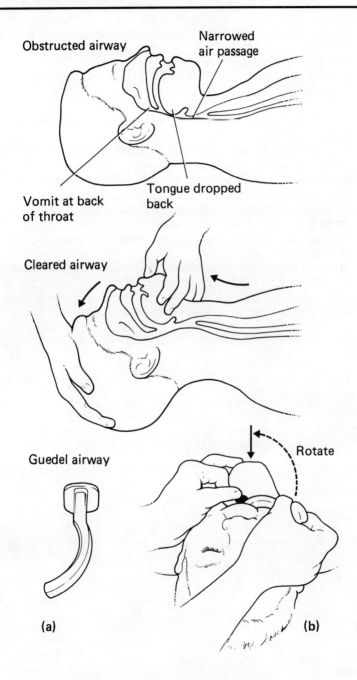

Obstructed airway

Narrowed
air passage

Vomit at back
of throat

Tongue dropped
back

Cleared airway

Guedel airway

Rotate

(a)

(b)

35 Suction

This is used to clear secretions from the mouth, pharynx and nose.

A   Suction equipment
B   Length of tube
C   The sucker (Yankauer type)

1   Ensure that you know how to work the suction unit before you ever have to use it.
2   Suckers come prepacked, and generally consist of a polythene tube attached to the sucker which is a plastic tube with an angled distal end. There is a hole in the back of the proximal part of the sucker, which allows a user to control the degree of suction by applying the thumb over the hole. The distal end of the sucker may have a series of small holes proximal to the opening, which prevent soft tissues, such as the uvula, being sucked into the sucker.
3   In an emergency situation where the sucker may be needed, turn it on and place the sucker below the pillow on the trolley. In this way, when the sucker is needed, it is readily available to clear the airway for intubation or the simple removal of secretions.

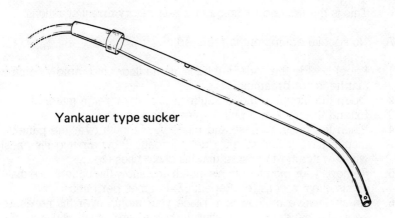

Yankauer type sucker

36 Mouth-to-mouth respiration

This is the first-aid technique for respiratory arrest situations.

A No special equipment is required

1 Kneel beside the patient, if he is on the floor, and rapidly confirm that he is not breathing.
2 Open the mouth, remove dentures and any foreign material.
3 Extend the neck and pull the jaw forwards (**a**).
4 Pinch the patient's nose and place your mouth over the patient's mouth, having first taken a deep breath. Blow air into his chest whilst watching to ensure that his chest rises (**b**).
5 Remove your mouth from his mouth and allow the patient to exhale as his chest recoils (**c**). Repeat 12–14 times per minute.
6 An alternative method is to place your mouth over his nose and keep the patient's mouth shut. In babies and small children, the resuscitator's mouth can be placed over both the child's mouth and nose.

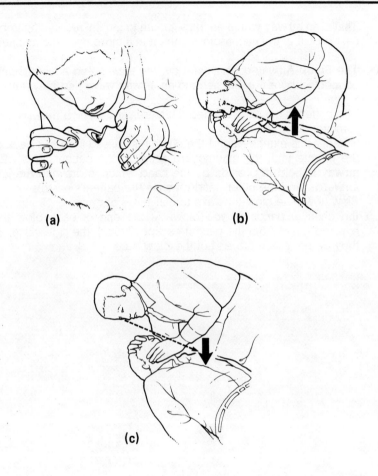

37 The Brook Airway

This is an airway which enables 'mouth to mouth' respiration to be carried out in the unconscious patient in a more hygienic manner.

A The Brook Airway consists of a curved airway and a mouthguard connected by a flexible neck to an airway valve and blow-tube

1 The patient's mouth is opened. Dentures and foreign material are removed from the mouth.
2 The head is extended and the airway is passed over the back of the tongue until the mouthguard rests on the patient's lips. The airway is held in position by the hand which is drawing the jaw forwards, and the other hand pinches the patient's nostrils.
3 Blow down the blow-tube at a rate of 12–14 per minute. Check that the chest expands as you blow. At the end of each blow the expired gases from the patient escape through the side valve, so they do not reach the end of the blow-tube.

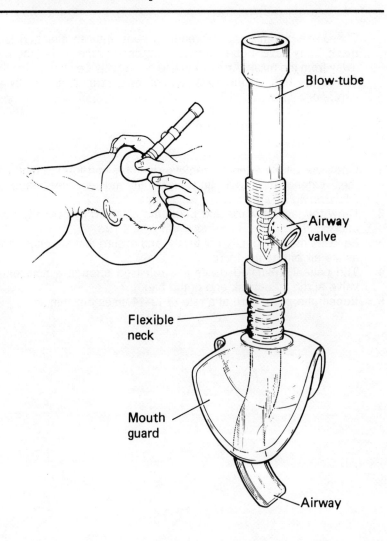

Blow-tube

Airway
valve

Flexible
neck

Mouth
guard

Airway

38 Bag and mask

These are self-inflating rebreathing bags with an attached face mask. They have a one-way valve attached to the end of the bag away from the mask. An oxygen line can usually be attached to this end of the bag. At the mask end of the bag there is usually an expiratory valve.

A   Bag and mask. Oxygen supply
B   Guedel Airway

1   Open the patient's mouth, remove dentures and foreign material, then extend the neck and insert an airway. (*see page 92 Maintaining an airway*).
2   Draw the jaw forwards and place the mask firmly over the nose and mouth.
3   Squeeze the bag gently but firmly, and ensure that the chest rises as the air enters the lungs.
4   The patient's exhaled gases are released through a non-return valve at the face-mask end of the bag.
5   Repeat the procedure at a rate of 12–14 times per minute.

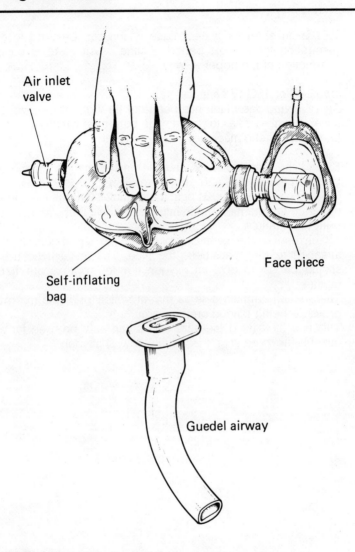

Air inlet valve

Face piece

Self-inflating bag

Guedel airway

39 Crico-thyroid stab

This is an emergency technique which can be used to obtain respiration for a short period of time when there is complete obstruction of the upper airway.

A Two 14G or 12G IV cannulas
B An IV giving set which has been cut through at the level of the lower chamber so as to give a wide bore tube which can be fitted to an anaesthetic machine

1 Extend the patient's neck, and feel in the midline for the space between the thyroid and cricoid cartilages.
2 Clean the skin, and insert both the cannulas through the midline of the crico-thyroid membrane into the trachea. Remove the needles from the cannulas.
3 Attach one of the cannulas to the giving set which should be attached to the anaesthetic machine. The anaesthetic machine should be set to give an oxygen flow of approximate 10 ℓ per minute.
4 The second cannula acts as a vent which prevents too great a pressure being placed on the lungs.
5 This is a life-saving measure and it can only be used for a few minutes, as there is an inadequate flow of oxygen.

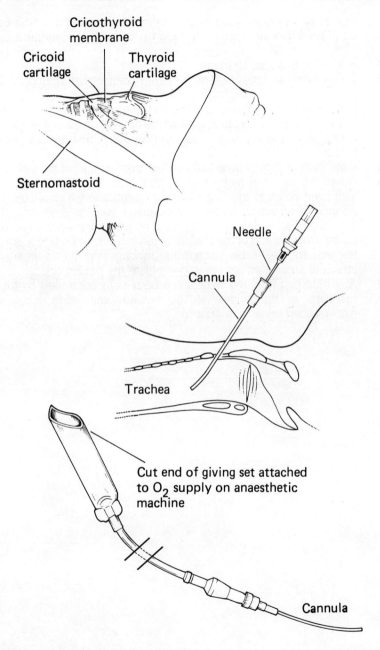

Cricothyroid
membrane

Cricoid
cartilage

Thyroid
cartilage

Sternomastoid

Needle

Cannula

Trachea

Cut end of giving set attached
to O_2 supply on anaesthetic
machine

Cannula

40 Crico-thyroid intubation

This is an emergency procedure by which a small bore tube can be placed into the trachea through the crico-thyroid membrane.

A Scalpel with a size 10 blade
B A paediatric endotracheal tube of approximate size 3 mm or 4 mm

1 Extend the patient's neck and feel for the space between the lower border of the thyroid cartilage and the upper border of the cricoid cartilage in the midline. This overlies the Crico-thyroid membrane.
2 If the patient is conscious infiltrate this area with local anaesthetic.
3 Clean the skin and make a short transverse incision through the skin right down to the Crico-thyroid membrane which should be opened. If an artery forcep is available it can be opened in the wound and so widen the opening. If no artery forcep is available place the blunt end of the scalpel in the incision and rotate it. Place the endotracheal tube through the incision into the trachea and attach to an oxygen source and ventilate the patient (c).
4 Any bleeding from the wound can be initially controlled by local pressure to the edges of the wound, until such times as experienced assistance arrives.

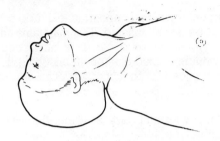

Cricothyroid membrane

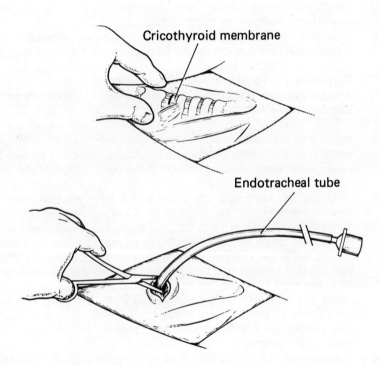

Endotracheal tube

41 Endotracheal intubation

This is a technique by which an endotracheal tube can be passed into the trachea and its cuff inflated. This maintains an airway and protects it from vomitus, blood etc. It is envisaged that, in an emergency, it would be used only on an unconscious patient and there would be no need for induction agents to put the patient to sleep, or for relaxants to paralyse the patient.

A   Endotracheal tube with cuff. Size 9–10 mm for adult male. Size 7–8 mm for adult female
B   A syringe to inflate the cuff of the endotracheal tube
C   The necessary connections to connect the endotracheal tube to an anaesthetic machine or to an Ambubag
D   A suction catheter with the suction checked and working
E   A malleable director, which can be placed down the endotracheal tube to alter its curvature
F   Tapes to tie the endotracheal tube in place
G   A laryngoscope that works. Check the bulb is secure and the batteries are fresh

1   Open the patient's mouth, remove dentures and suck out any vomitus or secretions. Place a pillow under the head so that the patient's neck is flexed, then extend the head on the flexed neck (**a**).
2   With the left hand, slip the blade of the laryngoscope over the back of the tongue to its full length (**b**). Gently lift the laryngoscope forwards, taking care not to trap the patient's lower lip and not to wedge the laryngoscope backwards in case the patient's upper incisor teeth are chipped or broken. The vocal cords should be visualized at this point. If there are any secretions suck them out.
3   With the right hand, slip an endotracheal tube of the correct size along the side of the laryngoscope blade, and pass the tube between the patient's vocal cords (**c**). A better view of the cords can be obtained with an assistant pressing on the larynx and pushing it upwards.
4   Inflate the cuff on the endotracheal tube until there is no audible air leak (5–10 ml), connect the tube to an oxygen supply and commence ventilation.
5   Tie the endotracheal tube in place after checking that both sides of the chest inflate equally. If the tube is passed too far it will enter the right main bronchus.
6   If visualization of the cords is difficult, or the tube cannot be passed between the cords because it is not curved enough, place the malleable director in the tube to change the curvature.

41 Endotracheal intubation

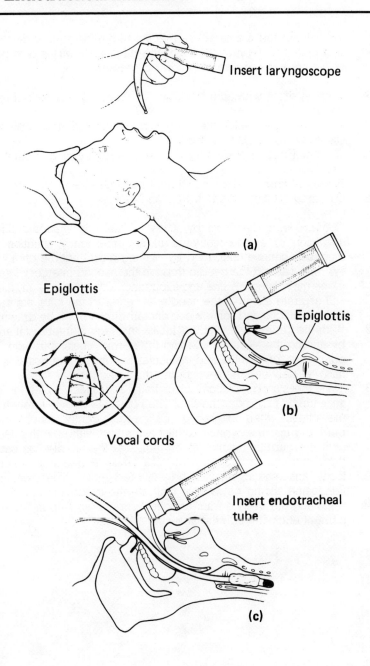

Insert laryngoscope

(a)

Epiglottis

Epiglottis

Vocal cords

(b)

Insert endotracheal tube

(c)

42 Chest drainage

This allows the drainage of air or fluid from the pleural cavity, so reducing the pressure placed on the lungs. It allows the restoration of the normal negative intrathoracic pressure.

A   A chest drain with an introducer, 24 French gauge to 32 French gauge

B   An underwater seal bottle with the right connections and 500 ml of sterile water to place in the bottle

C   15 ml of 1 per cent plain lignocaine in a 20 ml syringe with a 21G needle

D   A scalpel and 2/0 silk on a straight hand needle

E   Cleaning solution, sterile towels and gloves

1   Confirm your diagnosis by X-ray. If there is a strong clinical suspicion of a pneumothorax in an emergency situation, the diagnosis can be confirmed by placing a 21G needle on a 10 ml syringe, passing the needle through the second intercostal space in the mid-clavicular line and aspirating. If there is free air, the air will aspirate easily. If the needle has entered the lung, aspiration will be difficult and some blood and air bubbles will be drawn up.

2   With the patient lying supine, locate the second intercostal space by finding the sternal angle and the second costal cartilage. The point of entry is in the mid-clavicular line in the intercostal space midway between the second and third ribs (a).

3   Take the syringe of local anaesthetic and inject a bleb of local anaesthetic just under the skin. Then push the needle through into the chest, when aspirating the needle gently should cause bubbling into the syringe. Whilst aspirating withdraw the needle until the bubbling stops, which indicates the needle has passed through the parietal pleura. This is a sensitive area and 4 ml of the local anaesthetic should be injected now. The remaining lignocaine should be used to infiltrate the intercostal muscle. On removing the needle from the chest scratch an X to indicate the point of entry through the anaesthetized area (b).

42 Chest drainage

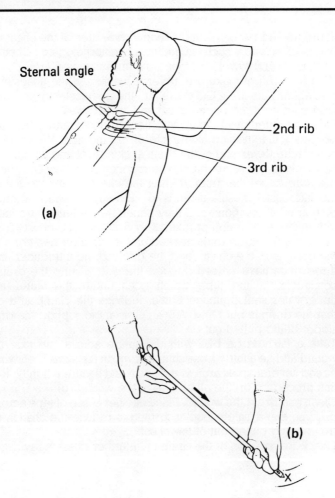

Sternal angle

2nd rib

3rd rib

(a)

(b)

4   Scrub-up and put on gloves. Clean a wide area of the chest with a coloured solution such as iodine or chlorhexidine. Check the landmarks and towel up around the anaesthetized area.

5   With the scalpel make a transverse incision in the anaesthetized skin about 1 cm long. Cut down into the intercostal muscle and do not be afraid if the pleura is cut and air escapes.

6   Take the intercostal drain with its introducer and place it in a perpendicular fashion at the site of the incision. With one hand control the lower end of the drain at skin level and with the other hand place pressure on the introducer. It takes considerable pressure to get the drain to enter the chest. As it passes through the intercostal muscle it tends to suddenly 'give' and it must be restrained at this point or it may penetrate the lung. Introduce the introducer and drain approximately 5 cm into the chest (past the middle of the three rings marked on the drain). When certain that the drain is in the chest, feed the drain off the introducer until all three rings have passed through the skin. Clamp the drain and connect it to the tube which goes under the water in the underwater seal drainage bottle. Release the clamp and check that the drain is bubbling. Ask an assistant to support the drain to stop it being pulled out.

7   Take a fairly large bite with the suture across one side of the wound and tie a fairly loose suture down on the skin. Then wind the thread several times around the drain and secure it tightly. Repeat this procedure on the other side of the wound (c).

8   Clean and dress the wound. Place another piece of tape across the drain so that a 'safety loop' is formed to reduce the chance of the drain being pulled out of the chest.

9   Check the position of the drain on a further chest X-ray.

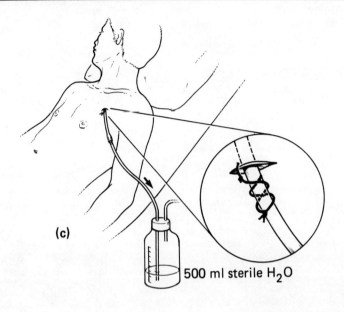

(c)

500 ml sterile H$_2$O

Section 4
Cardiac procedures

43 External cardiac massage

This is used in conjunction with ventilation to maintain a circulating volume of oxygenated blood in the cardiac arrest situation.

A   No special equipment is required

1   Someone must look after the airway and provide oxygenation.
2   The patient must be on a hard surface, such as a trolley, or if in a bed, a board should be placed below their back.
3   Place the heels of the hands over the lower sternum and depress the sternum approximately 5 cm, then release the pressure. This should be continued at an approximate rate of 60 per minute. The arms should be kept straight.
4   There is no need to stop external cardiac massage for the purposes of ventilation, as it is probably more beneficial in terms of gas exchange when the patient is ventilated against a resistance.
5   Another member of the team should check that there is a femoral pulse, indicating that massage is being carried out adequately.
6   Ventilation and external massage should be maintained in a continuous fashion as long as the patient does not have a cardiac output. It should not be started and stopped to allow deliberation. It is obviously stopped during defibrillation.
7   Excessively enthusiastic external cardiac massage will fracture ribs, and the rib ends can rupture the heart. In the case of babies, external cardiac massage can be carried out by placing the hands around the chest and the thumbs over the lower sternum. The rate must be increased to approximately 80 per minute and the pressure modified so as not to cause internal injury.

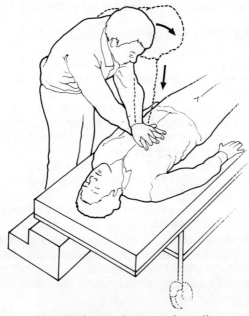

Remember — Ventilation and external cardiac
massage must be carried out together

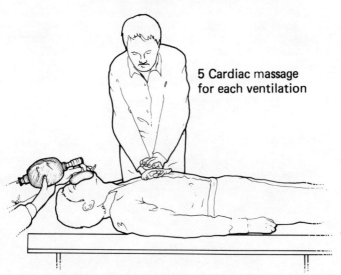

5 Cardiac massage
for each ventilation

44 Defibrillation

Cardiac defibrillation is carried out for ventricular fibrillation.

A A defibrillator with which you are familiar
B Electrode jel or pre-packed jel pads

1 Rapidly confirm the diagnosis of ventricular fibrillation from the monitor screen. Charge the defibrillator to 200 joules.

2 Place one electrode below the right clavicle just lateral to the upper sternum, and place the other electrode just lateral to the left nipple in the anterior axillary line. Ensure good contact with the electrode pads or jel and the skin.

3 Instruct everybody to stand clear of the patient and trolley, check that you are not touching the trolley and discharge the defibrillator through the patient.

4 The ECG trace on the monitor will be very irregular for a few moments before the definitive trace can be determined. Ventilation should be continued immediately after defibrillation and if there is any doubt about the resumption of sinus rhythm, cardiac massage should be continued.

5 If further defibrillation is indicated, the energy should be increased to 400 joules.

44 Defibrillation

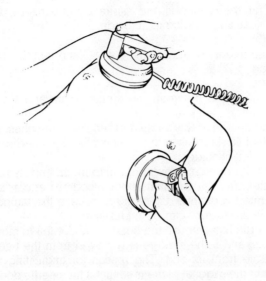

45 Pericardial tap

This is for the diagnosis and aspiration of a haemopericardium which is causing cardiac tamponade.

A   A cardiac needle of approximately 18G and length 10 cm
B   A syringe

1   Locate the angle between the xiphisternum and the left costal margin. Clean the skin.
2   Place the needle at this angle and run it into the chest upwards at an angle of 45 degrees to the horizontal and in the direction of the tip of the left shoulder.
3   Advance the needle through the diaphragm and gently aspirate. As it enters the pericardium either blood or pericardial fluid will be aspirated. Continue aspirating to relieve the tamponade until such time as surgery can be undertaken.
4   If the needle has entered the heart, it will be felt to move with the pulsations, and if the syringe is removed from the needle, blood will pulsate from its end. The reason for angulating the needle away from the saggital plane is so that if the needle does enter the heart it should enter the ventricle which will seal in a more satisfactory manner than the thin walled atrium would do, if it were penetrated.
5   If the needle does locate a tamponade, then the possibility of introducing a large bore catheter over a guidewire which can be inserted down the needle should be considered. This would then eliminate any hazards the needle might present to the heart.

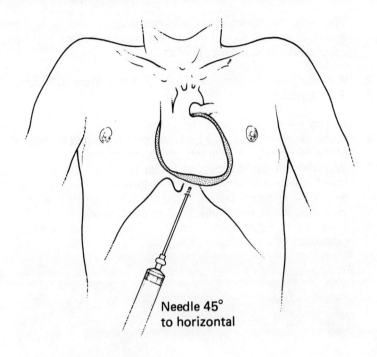

45 Pericardial tap

Needle 45°
to horizontal

46 Intracardiac injection

This is for the direct injection of drugs into the heart, in a cardiac arrest situation. It should only be used as a last resort and if there is no central venous line in position.

A   A cardiac needle (approximately 18G and 10 cm in length)
B   A 5 ml syringe

1   Locate the 4th left intercostal space
2   Place the needle midway between the nipple and the lateral edge of the sternum in the 4th left intercostal space.
3   With the needle in a perpendicular position, push it through the chest wall to its full depth, then withdraw and gently aspirate until a free flow of blood occurs. The needle should be in a cardiac chamber at this point. Inject the relevant drugs.
4   If resuscitation has been successful, X-ray the chest to exclude the possibility of a pneumothorax.

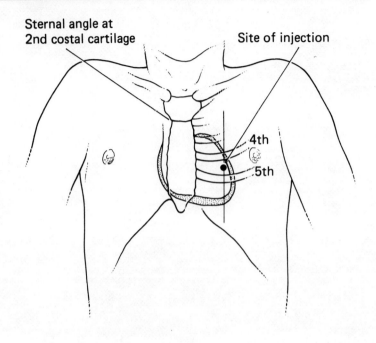

Sternal angle at
2nd costal cartilage

Site of injection

4th

5th

Section 5
Abdominal
procedures

47 Rectal examination

This permits the visual examination of the anus and it is followed by palpation of the lower part of the rectum. It is a mandatory part of every abdominal examination.

A   'PR' tray containing
(a) Disposable examination gloves of an appropriate size
(b) Lubricating jelly
(c) Paper or gauze wipes

1   Ask the patient to remove his underclothing, and to lie on his left side with knees drawn up to the abdomen (a).
2   Explain exactly what you are going to do. Tell the patient that it is an uncomfortable examination. If you are seeking for tenderness explain that this must be greater than the discomfort of the examination.
3   Lubricate the index finger of the gloved right hand. Draw the patient's buttocks apart with the left hand and place the right index finger against the anus, with the finger pointing in the direction of the patient's front. Gently press on the anus (b) until the anal sphincter gives and gently insert the finger into the rectum.
4   Examine the posterior wall of the rectum which is the hollow of the sacrum and coccyx, then examine the right lateral wall and check for discomfort (as can occur in appendicitis), check the left lateral wall, and then rotate the finger to examine the prostate in the male or the cervix in the female. Movement of the cervix may cause abdominal discomfort when the fallopian tubes are inflamed.
5   When you are satisfied that there are no other lesions to be felt, and you have checked the consistency of the faeces in the rectum, gently remove the finger and examine it for traces of blood and the colour of the faeces.
6   Gently clean the anal area of the patient with a wipe.

47 Rectal examination

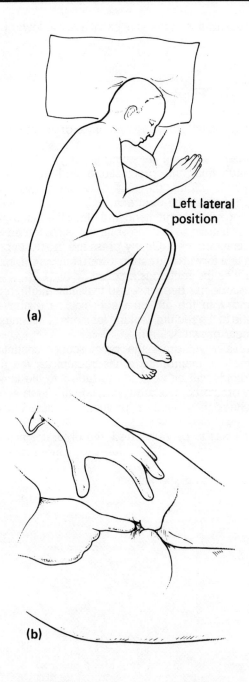

Left lateral
position

(a)

(b)

48 Proctoscopy

This allows the visualization of the anal canal and the lower part of the rectum.

A   A 'PR' tray (*see page 124*)
B   A disposable proctoscope
C   A light source

1   Place the patient on his left side, and ask him to draw his knees up to the abdomen.
2   Explain to the patient what you are going to do.
3   With gloved hands take the proctoscope and apply a little lubricating jelly to it, wiping the jelly over the outside of the proctoscope and the tip of the obturator.
4   Hold the proctoscope in the right hand and place the thumb on the top of the obturator handle so that the obturator is not forced out as the proctoscope is introduced. Gently press the proctoscope into the anus, starting in a forward direction towards the umbilicus, but turning posteriorly as the rectum is entered.
5   When the proctoscope has been inserted to its full length, remove the obturator, and with the aid of a light source examine the mucous membrane of the rectum, looking for signs of inflammation, ulceration or tumour growth.
6   Gently and gradually withdraw the proctoscope, continuously examining the mucous membrane of the rectum as you do so. Internal haemorrhoids will be seen to protrude into the lumen of the rectum as the proctoscope is drawn through the internal end of the anal canal, check their number, position and size. Withdraw the proctoscope.
7   If the proctoscope has to be reinserted, the obturator has to be replaced in the proctoscope and the whole procedure repeated as above.
8   Wipe clean the anal area of the patient.

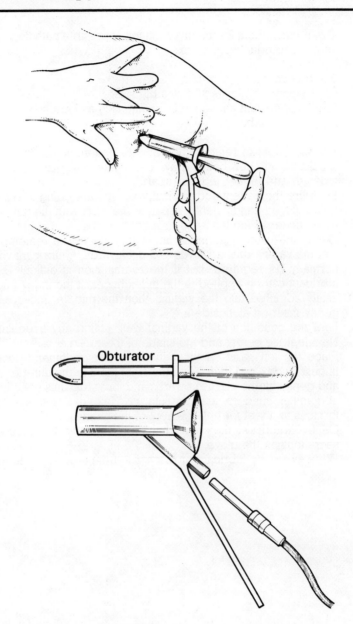

Obturator

49 Vaginal examination

This is carried out for the investigation of possible pathology in the female reproductive organs.

A 'PV' tray containing:
   (a) Disposable gloves of a suitable size
   (b) A non-irritant antiseptic lubricant such as Phisohex
   (c) Gauze swabs

1 Ask the nurse to remove the patient's underclothes. The patient should lie on her back, draw her knees up, place her heels together and let her legs fall apart.
2 Reassure the patient and explain what you are going to do.
3 Using gloved hands, gently separate the labia with the thumb and index finger of the left hand. Inspect the labia.
4 Gently insert the right index finger into the vagina remembering that the vagina runs upwards and backwards. A lubricant will not normally be required, but if the examination is difficult, a little lubricant can be applied to the index finger. If the index finger is easily admitted into the vagina, then the middle finger can be gently inserted alongside it.
5 Feel the condition of the vaginal wall, noting any irregularities. Next feel the cervix and the shape of the external os.
6 Place the left hand on the patient's lower abdomen. Place the fingers (index and middle) of the right hand in the anterior fornix and gently lift the uterus upwards and forwards, thus enabling the abdominal hand to feel the uterus. Next examine the lateral fornices and feel for enlargement of the ovaries.
7 Gently withdraw the right hand, and check for blood and secretions on the glove.
8 Wipe away any lubricant or discharge from around the labia.

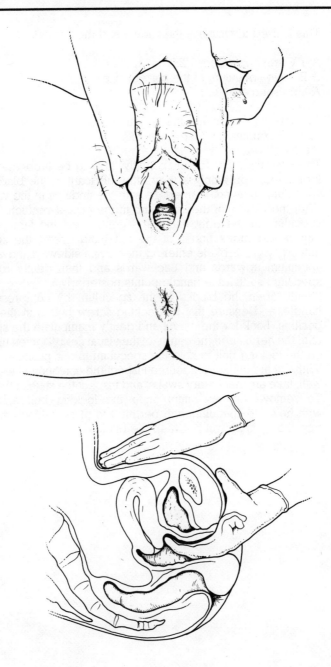

50 Speculum examination of the vagina

This is used to visualize the vagina and the cervix.

A A 'PV' tray. (*see page 128*)
B A Bivalve speculum of the correct size
C A light source

1 Ask the nurse to place the patient in the same position as for a vaginal examination (*see page 128*).
2 Put on gloves.
3 The speculum should not normally have to be lubricated. If it is lubricated, apply only a very little lubricant to the blade of the speculum so as not to interfere with the findings in the vagina.
4 With the blades of the speculum in the closed position, hold the speculum in the right hand, and gently part the labia with the thumb and index finger of the left hand. Insert the speculum initially with the blade entering the vagina sideways, advance the speculum upwards and backwards and then gently rotate the speculum so that the handle points posteriorly.
5 Gently open the blades of the speculum by compressing the handle, and ensure that the locking screw bolt is in the correct position. Look for the cervix and gently manipulate the speculum until the cervix is in the centre of the visual field. Tighten up the nut on the locking bolt to hold the speculum in this position.
6 With the aid of the light source inspect the condition of the vaginal wall, take any necessary swabs, and inspect the state of the cervix.
7 To remove the speculum undo the locking bolt and gently withdraw the speculum and permit it to close, taking care not to trap the vaginal wall between the blades.

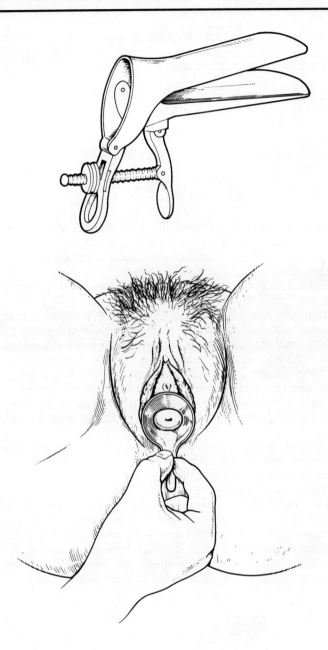

51 Male urethral catheterization

This is used to drain the bladder in cases of urinary retention, or in cases of major trauma where urine production is an indication of the patient's circulatory state.

A A bowl to collect urine
B Galley pots and woollen balls
C Sterile dressing sheets
D Sponge holding forceps
E A urinary catheter of between 14 and 18 FG
F A uribag to collect the urine
G An anaesthetic lubricant jelly
H 10 ml syringe and sterile water

1 Ask the nurse to remove the patient's clothing and place an incontipad under the patient's buttocks and between his legs.
2 Clean around the genitalia with a mild antiseptic solution such as Savlon.
3 Cut a hole in the centre of the sterile sheet and place it over the penis.
4 Tear the end off the plastic cover of the catheter, leaving the majority of the catheter inside the remainder of the cover. Apply a little anaesthetic jelly to the catheter tip. Ensure that you can reach the catheter easily when working with the patient.
5 If the patient is uncircumcised draw back the foreskin. Clean around the glans penis and the opening of the urethra. Hold the penis in your left hand. Take the catheter inside its cover in your right hand, ensuring that you do not touch the catheter and insert it into the urethra, by feeding the catheter out of the cover. Pass the catheter almost to its full length, some resistance will be felt as it passes through the prostate. As the catheter enters the bladder urine will run back into the plastic cover.
6 Take a urine sample for culture at this stage.
7 Put 10 ml of sterile water with a syringe into the retaining balloon of the catheter, via the side arm provided on the distal end of the catheter. Gently withdraw the catheter until the balloon just catches on the wall of the bladder. Now attach the catheter to the uribag, remove the sterile sheet, and ensure that the patient is clean and dry. Pull the foreskin forward if appropriate.

51 Male urethral catheterization

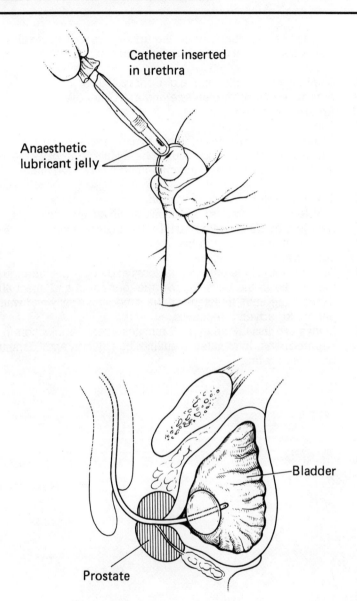

Catheter inserted in urethra

Anaesthetic lubricant jelly

Bladder

Prostate

52 Intravenous urography (IVU or IVP)

This is used to demonstrate the urinary tract. It is of value in the diagnosis of urinary calculi and in cases of possible renal trauma.

A 40 ml of contrast medium, e.g. Conray 480
B A syringe of appropriate size and a 21G needle
C An arm tourniquet
D Spirit to clean the skin
E 10 mg chlorpheniramine, 200 mg hydrocortisone, and 1 ml of 1:1000 adrenaline. These drugs should be available in case the patient has an anaphylactoid reaction to the contrast medium.

1 Take a history from the patient to exclude allergies, renal problems or possible conditions such as myelomatosis. These people may be placed at risk by the investigation.
2 Take a straight X-ray of the abdomen specifying that it is for the 'renal tract'.
3 Select a vein in the ante-cubital fossa and apply the tourniquet. Put the needle in the vein, remove the tourniquet and inject 40 ml of contrast medium. Inject the contrast medium slowly and watch the patient for adverse reactions.
4 X-rays are usually taken at 5 minutes after the injection to show nephrograms, 10 minutes to outline the calyces, and 20 minutes to show the ureters.

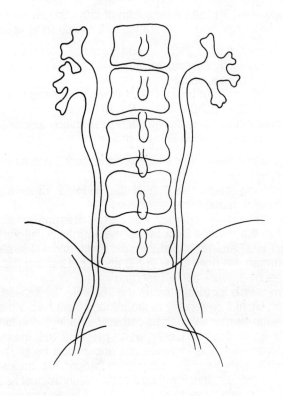

53 Peritoneal lavage

This is used for the investigation of intra-abdominal trauma which may have resulted in laceration of a viscus such as spleen, liver.

A Peritoneal dialysis catheter and trocar
B An intravenous infusion set
C 500 ml of normal saline
D 5 ml of 2 per cent lignocaine with a syringe and needle
E Size 3 scalpel handle with a No. 10 blade
F A basic dressing pack with skin preparation lotions
G A suture pack with a 2/0 silk suture

1 Catheterize the patient's bladder and gently press on the bladder to ensure that it is empty.
2 Thoroughly clean the skin of the patient's lower abdomen and shave abdominal hair if necessary.
3 Cover the lower abdomen with sterile dressing towels, leaving an area in the midline 5 cm below the umbilicus still visible.
4 Inject local anaesthetic at this site, first lifting a skin bleb and then infiltrating the linea alba. Try to avoid perforating the peritoneum as this may cause some bleeding.
5 Make a stab incision through the skin into the anaesthetized area which should be exactly in the midline 5 cm below the umbilicus.
6 Take the peritoneal dialysis catheter, and with one hand control it at the level of the abdomen, whilst pressing with the other hand on its upper end. The catheter and trocar must be perpendicular to the abdomen. As the trocar passes through the linea alba and into the peritoneum, there will be a sudden sensation of its giving. Care should be taken not to advance the catheter any further with the trocar. Advance the catheter off the trocar directing it to the right or left paracolic gutters.
7 Attach the saline and the intravenous infusion set to the catheter. Initially lower the saline bag below the patient and see if any blood can be siphoned from the abdomen at this stage. If this is negative, run 500 ml of saline into the abdomen and repeat the process of lowering the saline bag and siphoning back the saline.
8 A crude test for a positive result is if it is impossible to see newsprint through the siphoned fluid there is significant injury. If print can be seen but not read, significant injury is still probable.
9 A false positive result is possible if the introduction of the catheter has not been carried out with care.
10 After the saline has been siphoned back, the catheter can be removed and a suture placed in the abdominal wall.
11 The siphoned fluid is retained for laboratory investigation of its red cell content, and amylase estimation if pancreatitis is suspected.

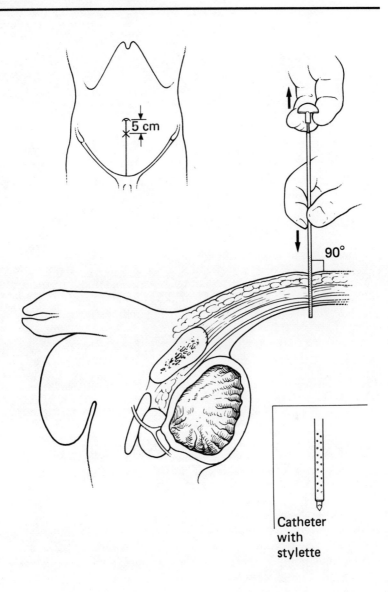

5 cm

90°

Catheter
with
stylette

Section 6
Local anaesthetic

For many procedures 1 per cent lignocaine will be adequate. It has a duration of action of about 60 minutes. For procedures where more time is required, then prilocaine in a suitable dilution may be more appropriate. In some procedures adrenaline (in a dilution of 1:200 000) may be added to the local anaesthetic. Adding adrenaline prolongs the anaesthetic effect and allows more local anaesthetic to be used. Adrenaline must *never* be used anywhere on the hand, foot, ears, nose or penis, as vasospasm of end arteries could be disastrous.

Where definite (maximum) quantities of local anaesthetic have been specified, these quantities are relevant to a 70 Kg adult patient. The quantities of local anaesthetic should be adjusted accordingly for smaller patients. The toxic dose for lignocaine is approximately 5 mg/Kg body weight.

55 Anaesthetic equipment

In all the techniques described in this section, it is necessary to draw up the anaesthetic solution into a syringe from either ampoules or rubber topped bottles using a 21G needle. Always check the details on the ampoule or bottle first. Clear the syringe of air before injecting anaesthetic. For techniques requiring only 1–2 ml of anaesthetic solution, a dental syringe is a convenient alternative.

In all the techniques described, at least a basic dressing pack or suture pack will be required. Hands should be thoroughly washed, and gloves should usually be worn. Gloves may not be necessary in simple procedures, where a no-touch technique can be used.

56 Wound infiltration

To allow thorough cleaning (debridement) and closure of a wound. Do not use on fingers and toes (use a digital block).

A   1 per cent lignocaine. (Maximum of 20 ml)
B   23G needle and an appropriate size syringe
C   Dressing or suture pack. Cleaning solution

1   Cover the wound with a gauze swab and clean a wide area of skin around the wound thoroughly with soap and water. (Use Swarfega if necessary.)
2   Gently clean the wound itself and the surrounding intact skin with the cleaning solution.
3   Push the needle through intact skin close to the wound edge, and inject local anaesthetic into the subcutaneous tissues in all directions. (Make sure that the needle is not in a vein or artery by withdrawing the plunger of the syringe before injecting.)
4   Make the second and subsequent injections from the edge of the anaesthetized area (in the same way as (3)) steadily working around the perimeter of the wound.
5   When all the injections have been made, wait a few minutes for the full anaesthetic effect.

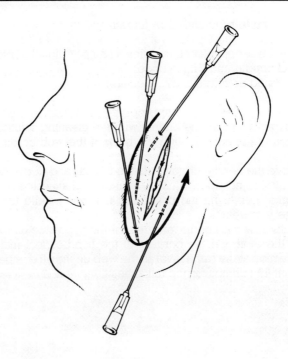

57 Digital block

For simple procedures on fingers and toes.

A   Use 1 per cent plain lignocaine. (1 ml per digital nerve is enough)
B   23G needle and 5 ml syringe
C   Dressing or suture pack. Cleaning solution

1   Clean the base of the appropriate digit, adjacent skin webs and surrounding skin thoroughly with the cleaning solution.
2   Push the needle through the back of the web on one side of the finger.
3   Move the needle tip towards the palmar and dorsal digital nerves in turn. Inject approximately 1 ml of local anaesthetic around each digital nerve, having confirmed that the needle tip is not in an artery or vein.
4   Withdraw the needle, and repeat the procedue on the other side of the digit. On the borders of the hand or foot make a second injection at the same level as the web on the other side of the digit.
5   Wait 10 minutes for the full anaesthetic action.

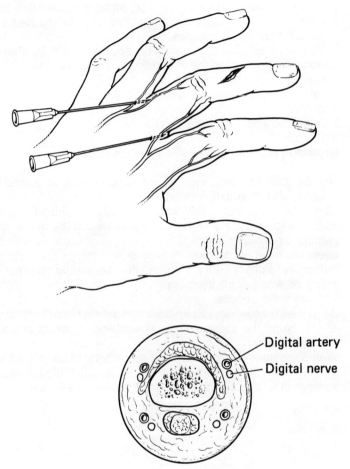

Digital artery
Digital nerve

Cross section at base of finger

58 Brachial plexus block (axillary approach)

For anaesthesia of the arm to allow (a) surgery on the hand, wrist or forearm, and (b) the application of a tourniquet during the surgery. It should work for 90 minutes.

The brachial plexus can also be approached from above the clavicle, in which case the circumflex nerve is also anaesthetized.

A 25 ml (maximum) of 1.5 per cent Prilocaine with 1:200 000 adrenaline
B 23G needle and 20 ml syringe(s)
C Tourniquet
D Dressing pack and gloves. Cleaning solution

1 Lay the patient down with the appropriate arm abducted to 90 degrees and externally rotated.
2 Clean the axilla thoroughly with the cleaning solution. Shave the axilla if necessary. Place the tourniquet around the upper arm.
3 Palpate the axillary artery.
4 Inject the local anaesthetic on each side of the axillary artery and behind the axillary artery. (Confirm that the needle tip is not in the artery or vein before injecting.)
5 Withdraw the needle.
6 Keep the arm elevated. Keep the tourniquet in place for 30 minutes as this helps the spread of the anaesthetic upwards around the brachial plexus.
7 Wait 30 minutes to allow the local anaesthetic to be fully effective. If a bloodless field is required then use an inflatable tourniquet to achieve this, after the anaesthetic has become effective.

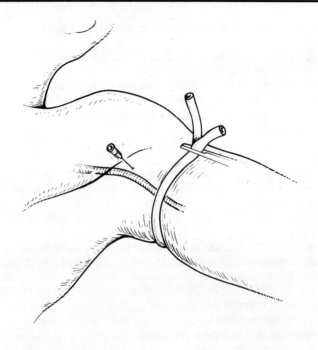

59 Regional intravenous block (Bier's block)

For manipulation of fractures in the wrist or hand.

A   A tourniquet, preferably double cuff but not automatic
B   23G needles and 20 ml syringes
C   40 ml of 0.5 per cent Prilocaine (for 70 Kg patient)
D   Esmarch bandage. Dressing pack, gloves and cleaning solution
E   Two people, one to perform the manipulation and one to supervize the tourniquet

1   Lay the patient down.
2   Place a 23G needle (Venflon or similar) in a vein of the non-operative arm. This allows quick venous access in an emergency.
3   Apply the tourniquet around the upper arm of the limb for manipulation.
4   Place a 23G needle in a peripheral vein of the same limb.
5   Elevate the limb and use the Esmarch bandage to exsanguinate the limb.
6   Inflate the tourniquet (proximal cuff) to 50 mm Hg above the patient's systolic blood pressure.
7   Inject the prilocaine through the needle ((4) above).
8   Remove the needle if required.
9   Wait for the anaesthetic to act before performing the manipulation (10–15 minutes). If using a double tourniquet, the distal cuff can now be inflated, and only then may the proximal cuff be released.
10   The tourniquet must remain inflated for at least 15 minutes even if the manipulation is completed earlier.

Complications

Reports of convulsions, cardio-respiratory problems and deaths due to the early release of local anaesthetic into the general circulation.

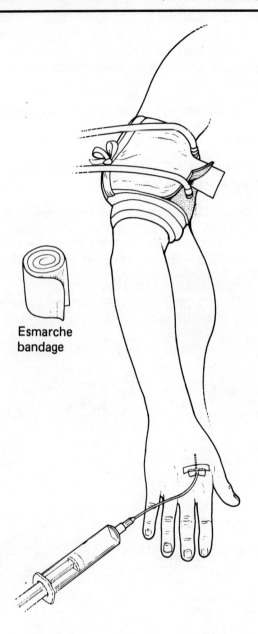

Esmarche
bandage

60 Femoral block

For pain relief in a fractured shaft of the femur. Together with a block of the lateral cutaneous nerve of the thigh, a femoral block anaesthetizes a large area of skin which can be used for donor grafting.

A 20 ml of 1 per cent lignocaine with 1:200 000 adrenaline
B 23G × 3.5 cm needle and 20 ml syringe
C Dressing pack, cleaning solution and gloves

1 Clean a wide area of the groin on the appropriate side thoroughly with the cleaning solution.
2 Palpate the femoral artery.
3 Push the needle to a depth of 3–4 cm immediately lateral to the femoral artery.
4 Check that the needle is not in the artery or a vein and inject the local anaesthetic in a fan-shaped distribution. Withdraw the needle.
5 Wait 20 minutes for the anaesthetic to act.

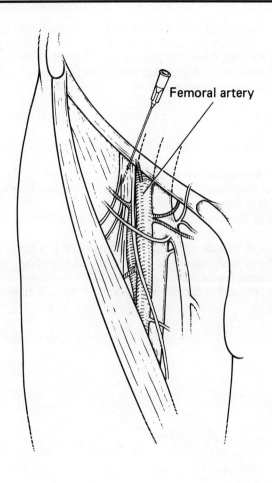

Femoral artery

61 Lateral cutaneous nerve of the thigh block

For anaesthesia of a skin area on the lateral side of the thigh, to allow moderate areas of skin to be taken for skin grafting. (It should only be used when the patient is unfit for general anaesthetic, and a moderate quantity of skin is required, as the skin grafting leaves a significant cosmetic defect.)

A   10 ml of 0.5 per cent lignocaine with 1:200 000 adrenaline
B   23G needle and 10 ml syringe
C   Dressing pack, cleaning solution and gloves

1   Have the patient lying down flat on his back.
2   Clean the skin of the groin out to the iliac crest thoroughly with the cleaning solution.
3   Identify the anterior superior iliac spine and find a point 2 cm along the inguinal ligament from here.
4   Push the needle through the skin below this point to a depth of 2 cm and inject the local anaesthetic in a fan-shaped pattern.
5   Withdraw the needle.
6   Wait 20 minutes for the anaesthetic to be effective.

61 Lateral cutaneous nerve of the thigh block

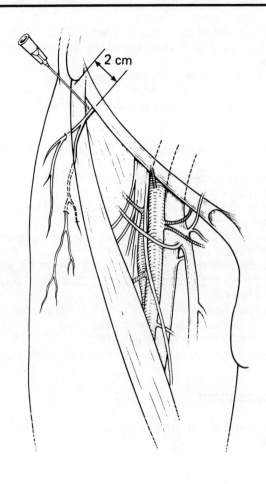

2 cm

62 Intercostal nerve block

For the relief of pain due to fractured ribs. It allows adequate physiotherapy and deep breathing. It should work for several hours.

A   5 ml of 1.5 per cent plain prilocaine
B   23G needle and 5 ml syringe
C   Dressing pack, cleaning solution and gloves
D   Marking pen

1   Sit the patient on the edge of a bed and lean the patient forwards over a table.
2   Identify the injured ribs by counting from the angle of the sternum (i.e. the second rib).
3   Mark points on the skin over the fractured rib(s) 8 cm from the midline posteriorly.
4   If the 4th and 5th ribs are involved, rotate the scapula forwards out of the way by elevating the arm.
5   Clean the skin thoroughly around the sites of the skin marks.
6   Push the needle through the skin at the mark to contact the lower part of the rib.
7   Adjust the needle direction and push the needle a further 3 mm inwards immediately below the rib.
8   Inject 5 ml of the local anaesthetic.
9   Withdraw the needle.

Complications

There is the possibility of a pneumothorax if the needle is pushed too far.

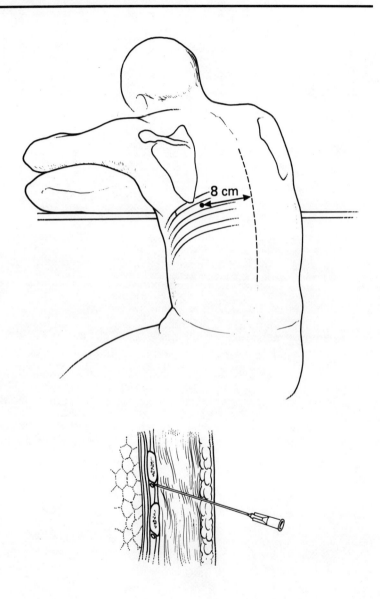

8 cm

Section 7
Minor surgical procedures

63 Ingrowing toenail

Wedge resection

For removal of excess granulation tissue and the damaged edge of
the nail.

A   Digital block (*see page 144*)
B   Rubber catheter as a tourniquet
C   Incision pack, cleaning solution and gloves
D   Steristrips

1   Anaesthetize the toe by digital block.
2   Clean the toe thoroughly.
3   Apply the tourniquet around the base of the toe, using strong
     artery forceps to hold it tight.
4   Drape the toe.
5   Using a scalpel cut a wedge of tissue from the affected side of the
     toe to include the edge of the nail. Extend the incision so that the
     wedge of tissue includes the root of the nail.
6   Use steristrips to gently close the resulting tissue defect.
7   Dress with paraffin gauze, melolin and tubigauze (or crepe
     bandage).
8   *Remove the tourniquet.*
9   The dressing should be changed after 7 days.

Note:

The remainder of the nail is left *in situ*. Removal of the whole nail
(avulsion) does not solve the patient's problem.

63 Ingrowing toenail

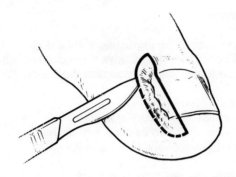

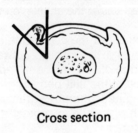

Cross section

64 Ingrowing toe nail

Phenolization

For the removal of the ingrowing toenail edge and the destruction of its nail bed. This is a definitive procedure which may be used in preference to the wedge resection (*see page 158*).

A Digital block (*see page 144*)
B Rubber catheter as a tourniquet
C Incision pack, cleaning solution and gloves
D 80 per cent phenol. Glycerine, alcohol

1 Anaesthetize the toe by digital block.
2 Clean the toe thoroughly.
3 Apply the tourniquet around the base of the toe, using strong artery forceps to hold it tight.
4 Drape the toe.
5 Cut a thin wedge of nail as indicated in the diagram (**a**). The cut must be continued *under* the cuticle to ensure the whole length of the nail is cut.
6 Place the forceps under the cut wedge of nail to the full length of their jaws and rotate the forceps outwards (**b**). Check that the whole of the wedge of nail has been removed, and a small piece has not broken off at the nail bed (**c**).
7 Curette the nail gutter to remove granulation tissue.
8 Coat the toe with glycerine to protect it from the phenol. Do not coat the nail gutter.
9 Place a small pledget of cotton wool, which has been soaked in 80 per cent phenol, under the cuticle and pack it into the corner of the nail bed. Leave for 3 minutes.
10 Remove the pledget of cotton wool, and scrape the exposed nail bed with the rough surface of one limb of a pair of non-toothed forceps.
11 Irrigate the nail bed and gutter well with alcohol.
12 Clean the toe, and dress with adhesive plaster. *Remove the tourniquet.* Check the colour of the toe.
13 Dressing instructions to the patient are 'to wear the plaster for 48 hours, then remove it at night, wash the toe and leave it exposed overnight. (The patient should use old bed linen.) Re-apply a fresh plaster each morning'. Review at 3 weeks.

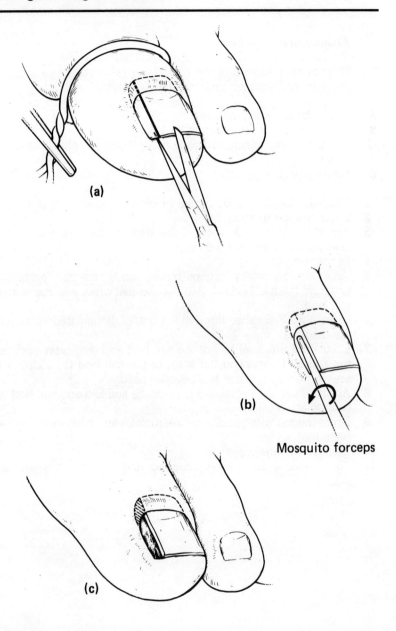

(a)

(b)

Mosquito forceps

(c)

Ablation of the nail bed

To prevent regrowth of the nail where there has been a chronic problem and simpler procedures have failed.

A Digital block (*see page 144*)
B Rubber catheter as a tourniquet
C Incision pack, cleaning solution and gloves, plus instruments described
D Suture material (4/0 silk)

1 Anaesthetize the toe by digital block.
2 Clean the toe thoroughly.
3 Apply the tourniquet around the base of the toe, using strong artery forceps to hold it tight.
4 Drape the toe.
5 Using straight artery forceps pushed under the nail, elevate the nail from the nail bed (**a**). Remove the nail when it is free from the nail bed.
6 Using a scalpel incise through the roof of the nail fold as shown in the diagram.
7 Excise the proximal half of the nail bed and the under-surface of the nail fold, including the sides of the nail bed (**b**). Curette the area from which tissue has been excised.
8 Approximate the remaining parts of the nail fold and nail bed with sutures (**c**).
9 Dress the toe with paraffin gauze, melolin and tubigauze (or crepe bandage).
10 *Remove the tourniquet.*
11 The dressing should be changed and sutures removed after 7 days.

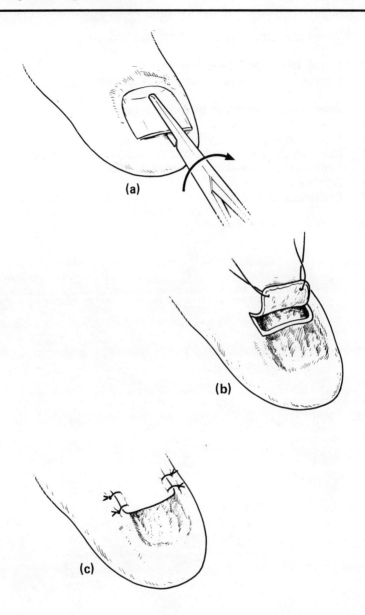

(a)

(b)

(c)

66 Paronychia, incision

When pus is present around the nail fold.

A   Digital block (*see page 144*)
B   Incision pack, cleaning solution and gloves

1   Anaesthetize the finger by a digital block.
2   Clean the finger thoroughly.
3   Drape the finger, by pushing it through a hole in a paper towel.
4   Make an incision over the pus in a longitudinal direction.
5   Remove the loose skin and expel the pus.
6   Apply a dressing.
7   Redress after 2–3 days.

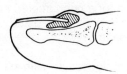

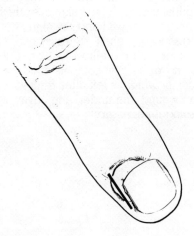

67 Sebaceous cyst excision

For the removal of a non-infected sebaceous cyst or implantation dermoid. If the cyst is infected and pus is present, then treat as an abscess (see page 174).

A 1 per cent plain lignocaine with syringe and 23G needle
B Suture and incision packs. Suture material

1 Clean the area around the cyst thoroughly. Shave hair as necessary around or over the cyst.
2 Inject the local anaesthetic through the skin into the subcutaneous tissues around the site of the cyst and deep to the cyst.
3 Make an elliptical incision in the skin over the cyst and define the plane between the cyst wall and the skin.
4 Using blunt dissection, 'shell' the cyst out. The cyst should be removed together with the ellipse of skin. If the cyst bursts, then continue to remove the cyst contents and cyst wall.
5 Curette the cavity which is left after removal of the cyst.
6 Close the skin wound and underlying cavity with sutures.
7 Apply a dressing if necessary.

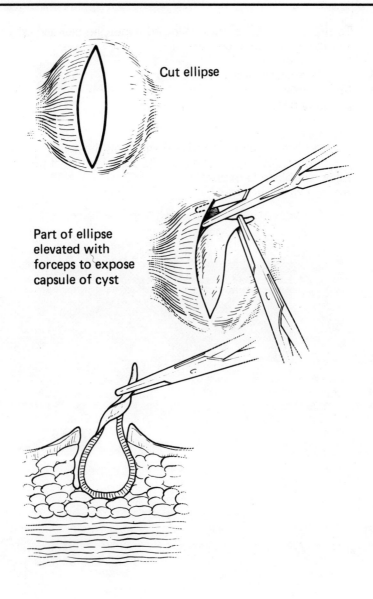

Cut ellipse

Part of ellipse
elevated with
forceps to expose
capsule of cyst

68 Subungual haematoma, drainage

To drain blood which has collected under the nail and which is causing moderate to severe pain.

A   Needle or straightened paper clip
B   Heat source
C   Dressing pack

1   Clean the nail.
2   Heat the needle or clip to red heat and apply the point to the nail. It will burn a hole through the nail with the minimum of pressure.
3   Allow the blood to drain.
4   Apply a small dressing.

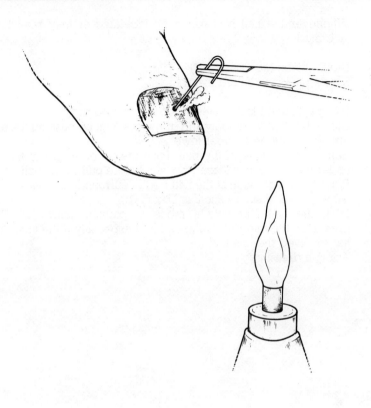

69 Injuries of the nail bed, repair

Whenever the nail bed has been lacerated or may have been lacerated.

A   Digital block (*see page 144*)
B   Suture pack and suture material

1   Using a digital block anaesthetize the injured digit.
2   Clean the digit thoroughly and drape the digit by pushing the digit through a hole in a paper towel.
3   Remove the whole of the nail. Push the tip of an artery forceps under the nail to fully loosen the nail, before pulling the nail off (**a**).
4   Repair any laceration of the nail bed or surrounding tissues with a 5/0 absorbable suture such as Dexon (**b**).
5   Pack the nail fold with a piece of paraffin gauze (**c**). (This preserves the integrity of the nail fold especially if the laceration has involved the nail fold.)
6   Apply a dressing.

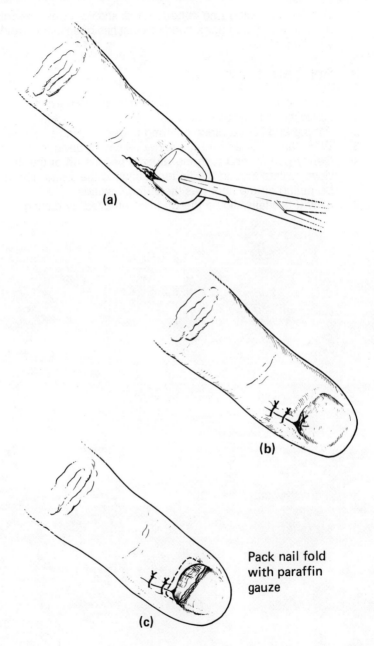

(a)

(b)

(c)

Pack nail fold
with paraffin
gauze

70 Ring removal

Try to avoid using ring cutters. Rings should always be removed from fingers if the finger, hand or wrist has been injured and tissue swelling is likely.

A   Soap, water and string.

1   Try first to remove the ring using soap and water to provide lubrication. If this fails then:

2   Put the end X of a piece of string under the ring as shown (**a**).

3   Wind the string around the finger as shown distal to the ring (**b**).

4   Gently pull on end X in the direction of the tip of the finger and slowly rotate around the finger to unwind the string. The ring will be pulled off the finger as the string unwinds.

5   Only if this fails should the ring be removed by cutting.

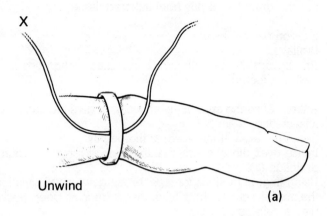

X

Unwind

(a)

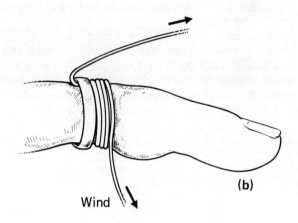

Wind

(b)

71 Abscess, incision and drainage

For the drainage of pus from infected tissue.

A   Incision pack. Gloves
B   Proflavin
C   An appropriate anaesthetic. (Local anaesthetic does not work as well in infected tissue)

1   Anaesthetize the area of the abscess, or give the patient a general anaesthetic.
2   Clean the area of the abscess thoroughly.
3   Incise over the abscess, making a good length incision to allow drainage (**a**).
4   Using fingers or sinus forceps, break down any loculations within the abscess cavity (**b**). Check that there is no deep pocket of pus (i.e., a collar stud abscess).
5   Pack the cavity lightly with gauze soaked in proflavin to achieve haemostasis. Use continuous gauze and leave the end of the gauze outside the cavity (**c**).
6   Apply gauze as a dressing over the pack.
7   See the patient the next day to remove the pack and apply a new dressing. Repacking should not normally be necessary. Change the dressings daily until drainage stops. Then keep the wound covered until the cavity closes.

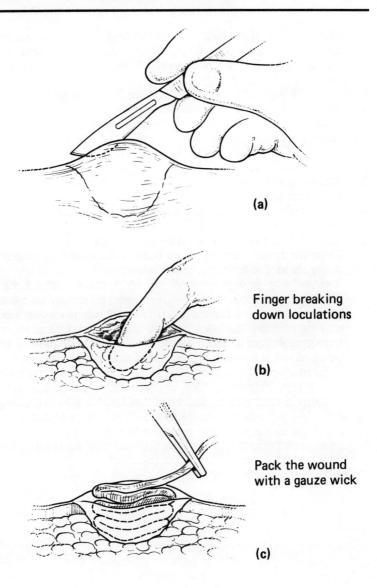

(a)

Finger breaking
down loculations

(b)

Pack the wound
with a gauze wick

(c)

72 Finger tip injuries (skin and bone loss): repair

The simplest procedure is often the best, in order to return the patient to work as soon as possible. Obtain expert advice if the patient needs fine discrimination for playing musical instruments, etc.

Skin defects of up to 1 cm diameter at the tip of the finger will heal without anything more than a protective dressing. Exposed bone will have to be covered by subcutaneous tissue to prevent future problems of pain.

A   Digital block (*see page 144*)
B   Suture pack
C   Bone nibblers
D   Silva's knife and blades for skin grafting (*see page 46*)

1   Anaesthetize the finger using a digital block.
2   Clean the finger thoroughly, and drape the finger by pushing the finger through a hole in a paper towel.
3   Remove any foreign material or dead tissue. Trim back any exposed bone until it can be covered with subcutaneous tissue. By careful nibbling of bone and excision of subcutaneous tissue, it may be possible to obtain primary skin closure by suture, where further slight loss of finger length is not important. The nail should be removed if the nail bed has been involved in the injury.
4   If the resulting skin defect is too large to heal by primary intention (i.e. >1 cm diameter), then apply a skin graft taken from the forearm. If the piece of skin which has been lost from the finger is available and relatively undamaged, then it can be used as a graft provided all the fat is first removed from it.
5   Dress with paraffin gauze, gauze and bandage. Remember to pack the nail fold if the nail has been removed.
6   Review at weekly intervals.

Exposed bone

Bone nibbled away
to give good soft
cover of tip

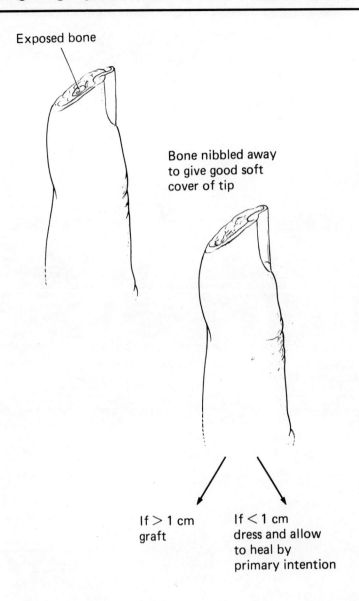

If > 1 cm
graft

If < 1 cm
dress and allow
to heal by
primary intention

Section 8
Bones and joints

73 The dislocated finger

For the reduction of a dislocated finger. Even if the finger has been reduced, X-rays should still be taken.

A   Digital block (*see page 144*)
B   X-rays
C   Tape for strapping or a Bedford splint

1   X-ray the dislocated finger to confirm the diagnosis and exclude any major fracture.
2   Anaesthetize the finger with a digital block.
3   Reduce the dislocation by applying traction and increasing the deformity, when the joint should be felt to click back into place.
4   Check that the joint is stable and the tendons function.
5   Take further X-rays to exclude small chip fractures around the joint which are indicative of ligamentous damage.
6   Strap the injured finger to the adjacent finger.
7   Warn the patient that the injured joint will remain swollen for several months.
8   If the joint is unstable or there appears to be ligamentous or tendon damage refer the patient for a specialist opinion.

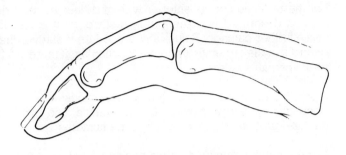

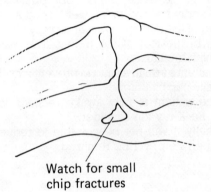

Watch for small
chip fractures

74 The dislocated shoulder

For the reduction of the anterior type of dislocated shoulder. The method described is a preferable method, as it is less likely to cause further damage. Before any procedure is started check and record that the circumflex nerve is functioning. If there is a fracture seek specialist help.

A   A suitable anaesthetic, usually a general anaesthetic
B   Good quality X-rays showing the dislocation, and excluding any fracture, particularly of the neck of the humerus

1   Lay the patient down flat on his back on a trolley.
2   Anaesthetize the patient.
3   Put a fist in the axilla of the appropriate shoulder or have an assistant apply traction to a towel looped around the axilla.
4   Take hold of the patient's wrist and apply traction on the arm in the direction of the foot of the trolley. The dislocation should now reduce with a clunk.
5   Put the patient's arm in a sling to prevent movement of the shoulder as he wakes up.
6   When the patient is fully awake recheck for circumflex nerve function. Re-X-ray the shoulder.
7   Occasionally it will not be possible to reduce the shoulder and more expert help will be required.

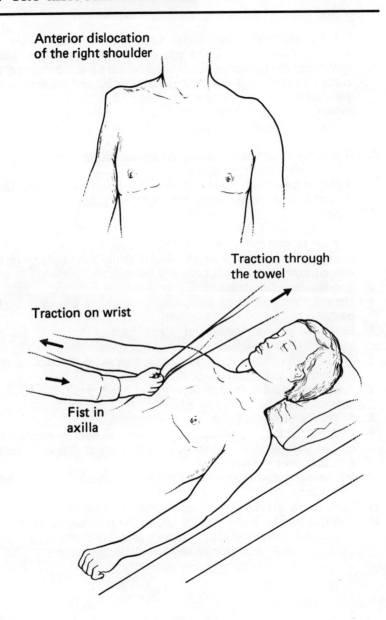

Anterior dislocation
of the right shoulder

Traction through
the towel

Traction on wrist

Fist in
axilla

75 The Colles's fracture

For the reduction of the Colles's fracture and the application of a suitable plaster slab. Good prereduction X-rays are required confirming the presence of a Colles's fracture (i.e. a fracture of the lower end of the radius with dorsal angulation and impaction) and the absence of other bony injury. A record should be made of the state of the circulation in the hand and the movements and sensation of the fingers before starting the procedure.

A   A suitable anaesthetic, usually a general anaesthetic. A regional intravenous block can be used
B   A plaster slab made out of a 20 cm POP roll as shown. Orthopaedic wool and stockinette. Cotton bandage (*see page 192*)
C   Sling

1   Lay the patient down flat on a trolley.
2   Remove all rings and other jewellery from the hand and arm on the injured side, if this has not already been done.
3   Anaesthetize the patient.
4   Have an assistant hold the patient's elbow to provide counter traction.
5   Hold the patient's hand and apply traction, to disimpact the fracture.
6   Whilst continuing to apply traction, first increase the angulation of the fracture and then reduce the fracture.
7   Apply the stockinette bandage to the hand, wrist and forearm, having cut a hole for the thumb.
8   Apply the orthopaedic wool over the stockinette.
9   Keeping the fracture reduced, apply the POP slab leaving the gap on the ventral side of the wrist and forearm. Apply a cotton bandage over the slab.
10 Put the patient's arm in a sling. Check the circulation of the hand is satisfactory.
11 Take check X-rays to confirm the position of the fracture.
12 There should be a check of the plaster the next day to ensure that there is no gross swelling of the fingers and the patient can move the fingers well with normal sensation and circulation.

75 The Colles's fracture

Disimpact and increase backward angulation

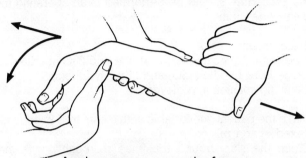

Apply pressure across the fracture
to obtain reduction

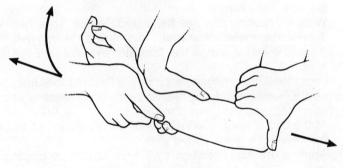

Plastering position

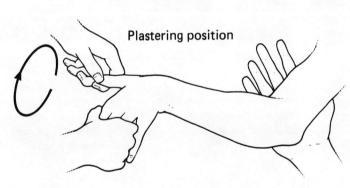

76 Knee aspiration

To remove fluid or blood from the knee joint, when there is a large effusion or haemarthrosis. Strict aseptic technique is required, and the procedure should be performed in an operating theatre, or a clean side-room.

A Basic dressing pack
B 1 per cent lignocaine, 5 ml syringe and 23G needle
C Large bore needle (18G) and 20 ml syringe(s)
D Cleaning solution and gloves

1 Make the patient comfortable with the injured knee resting slightly flexed over a pillow.
2 Clean the skin around the knee thoroughly with the cleaning solution, and then drape the knee with towels.
3 Infiltrate the skin above and lateral to the patella with about 2 ml of the local anaesthetic.
4 Without touching the needle, introduce the large bore needle through the anaesthetized skin, and push it inwards until it enters the suprapatellar part of the distended synovial cavity of the knee joint.
5 Using the 20 ml syringe(s) aspirate the fluid or blood from the knee joint. Check the volume of fluid removed. If there is any sign of infection, send fluid for culture.
6 At the end of the procedure perform a full clinical examination of the knee in its undistended state.
7 Apply a dressing, followed by a wool and crepe bandage to the knee.

Knee aspiration

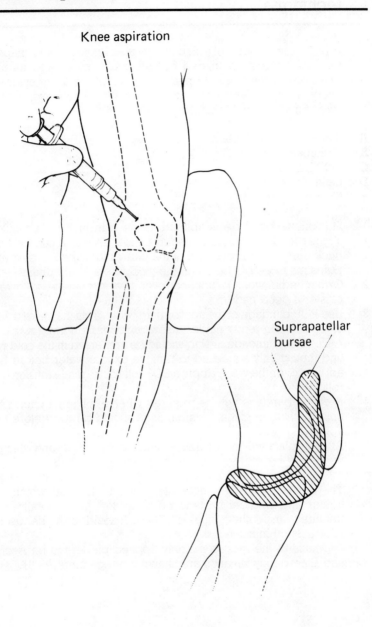

Suprapatellar
bursae

77 Basic plaster (plaster of Paris or POP) technique

A plaster in the form of a slab or completely enveloping shape can be used to rest an injured or inflamed joint as well as in the treatment of fractures. All plasters put on in the acute stage of an injury must be well padded to allow for the changes in tissue swelling which will take place.

A   Stockinette bandage
B   Orthopaedic wool
C   POP bandage
D   Cold water
E   Cotton bandage

1   Stockinette bandage is applied to the skin first. This should be slightly longer than the intended plaster so that it can be turned back during the application of the plaster to make a neater effect. Holes may need to be cut in the stockinette for the thumb etc.
2   Orthopaedic wool is applied over the stockinette to give the plaster a good padding.
3   Use POP bandage of the appropriate width. This may take the form of a roll or be ready made as several layers to form a slab.
      The POP bandage or slab should be immersed in the cold water and then gently squeezed to remove excess water before being applied over the wool. Apply a POP roll using gentle tension on the roll.
4   A cotton bandage will be required when applying a back slab to hold the slab in place. This bandage should be wet before being applied.
5   After application the plaster should be smoothed and shaped if necessary by rubbing and pressure with wet hands.

There are alternative materials available to POP which allow lighter and stronger casts to be made for the immobilization of fractures and other injuries. These should only be used in specialist circumstances.

Details of the most commonly applied plasters in an Accident and Emergency situation are shown in Procedures 78–81.

77 Basic plaster (plaster of Paris or POP) technique

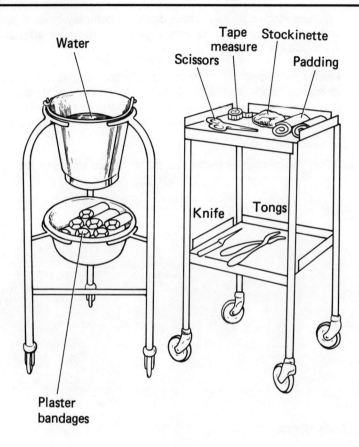

Water

Tape measure

Stockinette

Scissors

Padding

Knife

Tongs

Plaster bandages

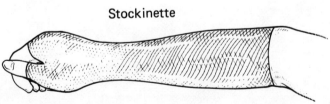

Stockinette

78 Backslab POP

This is a slab of plaster which does not completely envelope the limb. It can be used to rest a joint, or may be adequate to immobilize a fracture.

A   Plaster roll of suitable width which is folded on itself to make a slab of six or eight layers. POP slabs can be bought which are multi-layered and they only need cutting to length

B   Stockinette, orthopaedic wool, water and cotton bandage (*see page 188*)

1   Apply the plaster as instructed in the details on *page 188*.

Back slab POP as in Colles's fracture

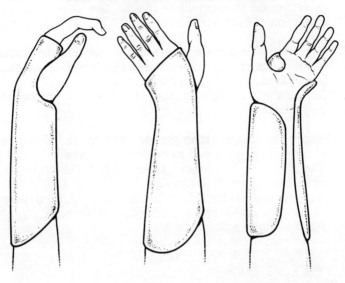

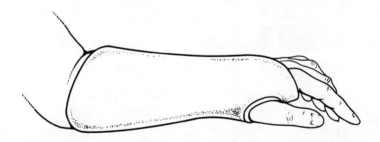

79 Colles's POP

This is initially applied as a backslab which after 24 hours or longer is converted to a complete plaster. See also *page 184* for the reduction of this fracture.

A A plaster slab is made to the shape shown in the diagram from eight layers of a 20 cm wide roll. The length of the slab should allow clear finger and elbow movements

B Stockinette, orthopaedic wool, water and cotton bandage (*see page 188*)

1 Apply the plaster during the reduction of the Colles's fracture as illustrated opposite, and as described on *pages 184* and *190*.

2 The plaster is completed subsequently by the further application of a 7.5 cm roll of POP bandage.

3 It is important to check the circulation, sensation and movements of the fingers, and to check for swelling in the hand.

4 Put the arm in a sling.

Dinner fork deformity

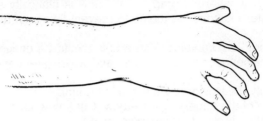

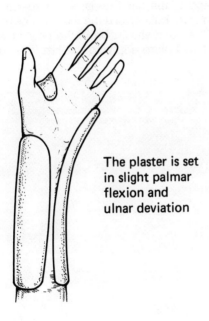

The plaster is set
in slight palmar
flexion and
ulnar deviation

80 Scaphoid POP

This should be applied for any scaphoid fracture seen radiologically or where a scaphoid fracture is clinically suspected. The plaster includes the thumb to prevent flexion of the thumb.

A 7.5 cm POP bandage. Three rolls should be enough
B Stockinette, orthopaedic wool and water (*see page 188*)

1 Apply the stockinette to the injured limb so that it covers from the base of the fingers to the elbow. Cut a hole for the thumb.
2 Apply a layer of orthopaedic wool.
3 Apply the POP bandage to the hand, wrist and forearm. Allow room for the fingers to move, but enclose the thumb to beyond the interphalangeal joint. The hand should be in the position shown. Fold the stockinette back, before applying the last layer of POP bandage.
4 Smooth the plaster.
5 Put the arm in a sling.

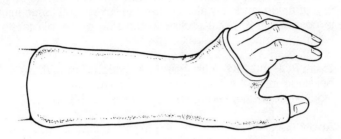

81 Below knee POP

This plaster can be used for the immobilization of fractures of the foot or ankle, and may also be used in severe soft tissue injuries. It is possible to apply a rocker to the sole of the plaster to allow weight bearing.

A   15 cm POP roll. Five rolls should be enough. One of these rolls may be made into a backslab which is applied first

B   Stockinette, orthopaedic wool and water (*see page 188*)

1   Apply the stockinette to the leg from the toes to the knee.

2   Apply adequate layers of orthopaedic wool especially around the ankle.

3   Apply a 15 cm POP backslab to the leg over the wool covering the sole of the foot, heel and calf.

4   Use the other rolls of POP to wrap around the limb enclosing the backslab. Leave the toes free and allow the knee to move fully. Whilst applying the plaster make sure the foot is held so that the ankle is in 90 degrees of dorsi-flexion. This is most easily achieved by pressing on the patient's toes with one's chest.

5   Turn back the stockinette before applying the last turn of plaster and smooth the plaster to give a neat finish.

6   If the patient is to walk on the plaster, then apply a rocker using a roll of POP to attach it to the plaster.

7   Watch the circulation and sensation of the toes, and check for swelling.

8   The patient will need crutches. Even if it is a walking plaster he will need to keep his weight off the foot until the plaster dries.

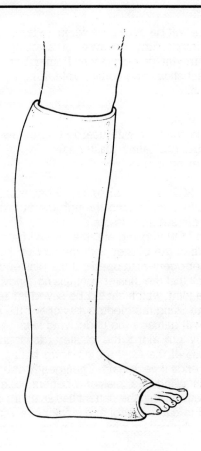

There will be occasions when a Plaster cast has to be removed as an emergency, because of swelling, severe pain or due to impairment of circulation. Remember that in a Plaster cast the patient should be comfortable. If he is in pain there is something wrong.

A   Plaster shears
B   Strong scissors, with guarded tip to lower blade
C   Electric oscillating plaster saw
D   Plaster openers

1   If the POP is incomplete as in a backslab, then it will be possible to remove it by cutting through the area where there is no plaster with the strong scissors.
2   If the POP is complete, then it will be necessary to cut along the length of the plaster with the saw or the shears, before using the plaster openers to open out the plaster so that it can be removed.
3   Check that the plaster contains no 'fancy' devices such as a hinged 'knee joint' which should be saved for reuse.
4   Before using the electric saw check the plaster is well padded, or you will damage the underlying skin.
5   Gently cut along the plaster (down the middle of the palmar surface of the forearm, or down both sides of the leg). Cut from both ends if necessary. Then gently open out the plaster with your hands using the plaster openers to make the initial opening. Remember that the patient has an injury under the plaster. You will need to cut the wool and stockinette with the scissors.
6   Splint the patient's injury as necessary.

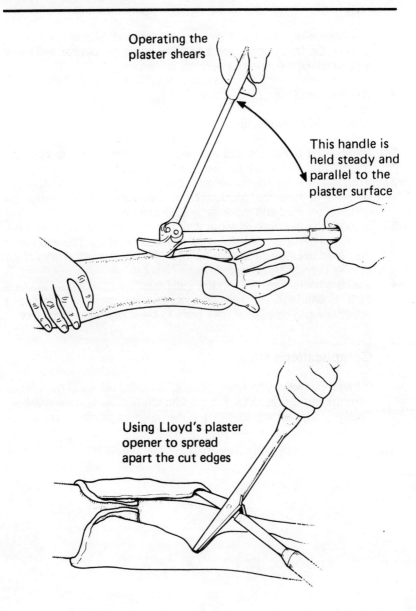

Operating the plaster shears

This handle is held steady and parallel to the plaster surface

Using Lloyd's plaster opener to spread apart the cut edges

Sometimes a patient will have very localized pain underneath a plaster. On these occasions a window cut in the plaster will allow inspection of the skin to check all is well.

A   Electric oscillating plaster saw
B   Scissors
C   A roll of POP and water

1   Identify the point at which you need to cut the plaster to view the underlying skin. Mark the window you wish to cut.
2   With the saw gently cut along the edges of the window. Use the scissors to free the window from the surrounding plaster, by cutting the wool and stockinette underneath.
3   Inspect the skin etc. If all is well the window can be replaced, provided there is adequate wool to act as padding. The window is then held in place by using a roll of POP to reinforce the area of the plaster containing the window.
4   If all is not well then the window can be either loosely held in place with a bandage, or removed completely to allow continuing observation. The plaster may have to be completely removed.

Complications

If there is inadequate wool padding, then the edges of the plaster surrounding the window will cut into the skin and cause damage. This will happen whether or not the piece of plaster is replaced.

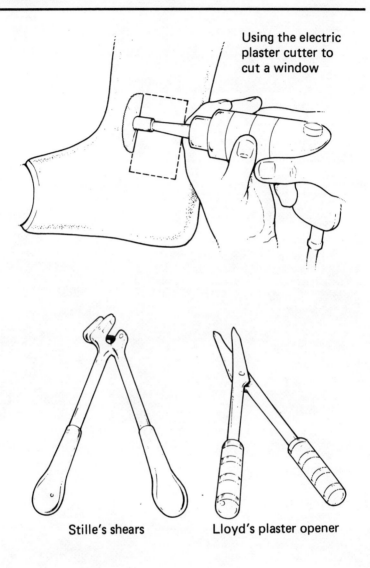

Using the electric
plaster cutter to
cut a window

Stille's shears   Lloyd's plaster opener

Section 8
ENT, Eyes and dentistry

84 Everting the eyelid

To allow examination of the under-surface of the upper eyelid and the superior fornix of the conjunctiva. It also enables foreign bodies to be removed from the same areas.

A   An orange stick

1   Ask the patient to gently close his eyes.
2   Grasp the eyelashes of the upper eyelid between finger and thumb.
3   Place the orange stick along the base of the upper eyelid (**a**).
4   Evert the eyelid over the orange stick (**b**) and then remove the stick (**c**).
5   At the end of the examination, ask the patient to blink, and the eyelid should fold back to normal.

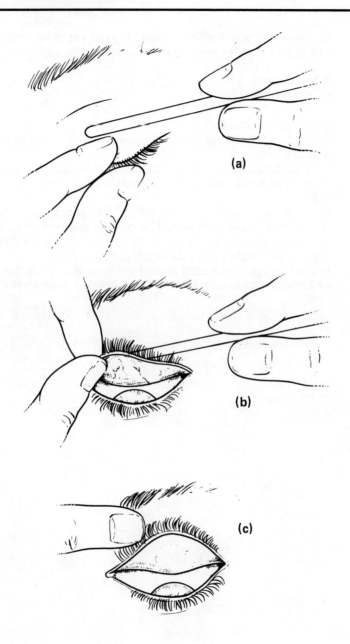

84 Everting the eyelid

(a)

(b)

(c)

85 Using the head mirror

To give good vision when looking into the ear, nose or mouth. It leaves both hands free to hold instruments etc.

A A head mirror
B A light source

1 Sit the patient down.
2 Fit the head mirror so that you can see directly through the hole with one eye.
3 Sit down facing the patient at a comfortable working distance, with the patient positioned so that you are looking at the appropriate orifice.
4 Place the light source to the side of the patient with the light shining at you. The light should be on the same side of the patient as the eye which looks through the mirror, i.e. your right eye = light on your right-hand side of the patient.
5 Adjust the light and mirror so that the light shines into the orifice which you wish to look at. Make sure you are comfortable.

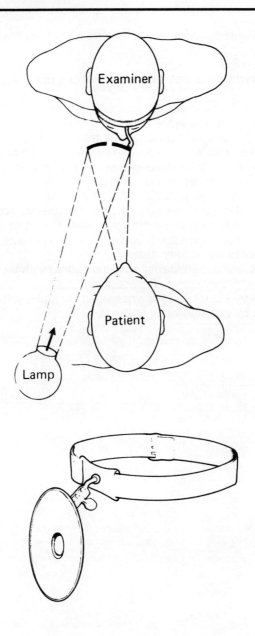

86 Syringing the ear

For the removal of wax or foreign body from the external ear.

A   Auriscope
B   Ear syringe, kidney dish and bowl of tepid water

1   Examine the external acoustic meatus with the auriscope to confirm the presence of wax or foreign body. Confirm that the patient has no history of a perforated eardrum.
2   Fill the bowl with tepid tap water at about body temperature.
3   Place the kidney dish against the patient's neck below the ear which is to be syringed.
4   Fill the syringe with water from the bowl.
5   Insert the tip of the syringe into the external acoustic meatus in such a way that, as the syringe is used, the water is directed along the roof of the meatus. The water and wax or foreign body should collect in the kidney dish.
6   Re-examine the external acoustic meatus with the auroscope, and repeat the syringing as necessary.
7   If the wax is too hard to syringe out, it can be softened over a few days by instilling suitable drops.

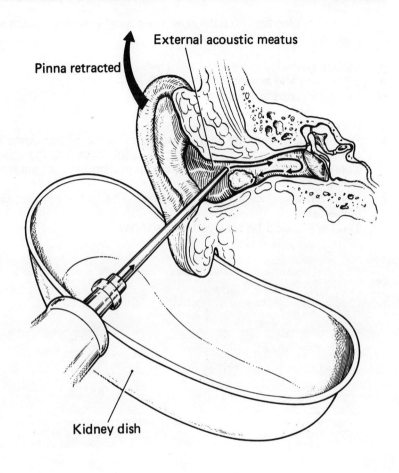

External acoustic meatus

Pinna retracted

Kidney dish

87 Packing the nose

To control bleeding from the nose when simple measures such as pinching the nose have failed.

A Ribbon gauze
B BIPP paste and a small bowl
C Heath's forceps or similar

1 Soak the ribbon gauze in BIPP paste.
2 Pack the nose from the floor upwards laying the ribbon down in layers, and using the forceps to push each layer into the nose. Keep both ends of the ribbon gauze protruding from the anterior nares.
3 If this packing does not stop the bleeding, ask for specialist help immediately.
4 The pack should be removed the next day.

87 Packing the nose

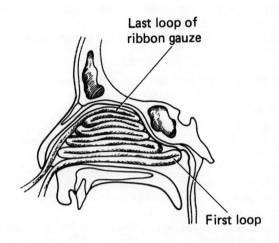

Last loop of
ribbon gauze

First loop

88 Cauterizing the nose

To prevent further bleeding from the nose, in a patient who has had a recent epistaxis, and where the bleeding point can be identified. The site of bleeding is usually Little's area on the septum.

A   A head mirror and suitable light source (*see page 206*)
B   Nasal speculum, and suitable forceps
C   Cotton wool
D   Solution of 4 per cent lignocaine and 1:1000 adrenaline
E   Electric cautery or 40 per cent silver nitrate solution

1   Soak some cotton wool in the lignocaine/adrenaline solution and use it to pack the anterior part of the nose for 5 minutes.
2   Remove this pack, and under direct vision identify the place from which bleeding has occurred.
3   Using the electric cautery or the silver nitrate solution, cauterize the bleeding point.
4   If this fails to control the bleeding then pack the nose (*see page 210*)
5   Remember to assess the whole patient and transfuse the patient if necessary.

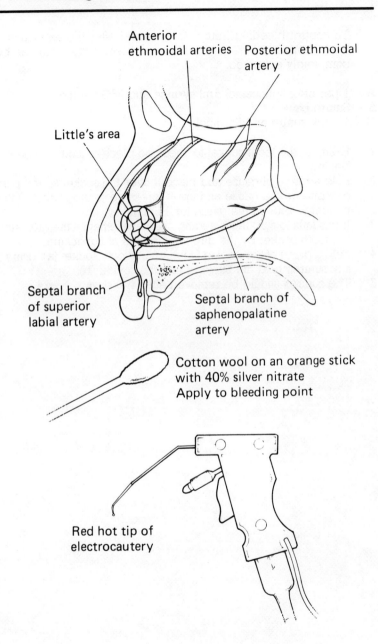

Anterior ethmoidal arteries

Posterior ethmoidal artery

Little's area

Septal branch of superior labial artery

Septal branch of saphenopalatine artery

Cotton wool on an orange stick with 40% silver nitrate
Apply to bleeding point

Red hot tip of electrocautery

89 The bleeding tooth socket

To control bleeding from a tooth socket after the extraction of a tooth. Normally bleeding is not a problem if the tooth has been completely extracted.

A 1 per cent lignocaine, 5 ml syringe and 25G needle
B Suture pack
C 4/0 silk suture and Surgicel

1 Examine the tooth socket to check no piece of tooth has been left behind.
2 Fold a piece of gauze and place it over the socket so the patient can bite on the gauze and apply pressure to the socket. Ask the patient to bite on the gauze for 10 minutes.
3 If this fails to stop the bleeding, then anaesthetize the gum around the tooth socket by the direct infiltration of lignocaine.
4 Fold a piece of Surgicel to fit the empty tooth socket (a). Using two silk sutures hold the Surgicel into the socket (b).
5 The sutures should be removed after 4–5 days.

89 The bleeding tooth socket

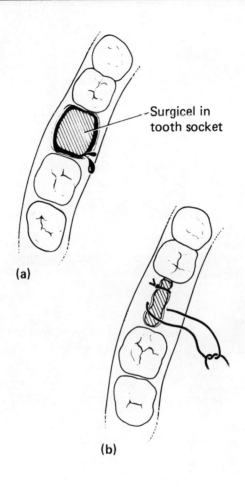

Surgicel in tooth socket

(a)

(b)

Section 10
Foreign bodies

90 Wound

For the removal of foreign bodies from wounds which are fresh or may have healed, and where the foreign body is *superficial* to the deep fascia. Not all foreign bodies have to be removed as their removal may cause more damage than leaving them *in situ*. Deep foreign bodies require a general anaesthetic and a bloodless field. However foreign bodies act as a focus for infection. Most glass shows on X-ray.

A Suitable anaesthetic
B Suture and incision packs
C X-rays may be helpful
D Patience

1 If it is suspected that a foreign body is present at the site of a wound, then take X-rays if the foreign body may be radio-opaque. If a foreign body is seen on X-ray then further films, with markers (paper clips) applied to the skin, may be helpful in locating it. Mark the site of the markers on the skin with an indelible pen.
2 Prepare the wound for wound closure with a suitable anaesthetic, and cleaning technique. If the wound has healed then incise over the site of the foreign body, after cleaning and towelling the skin.
3 Using the X-rays and markers as guides locate the foreign body and remove it.
4 Close the wound in the normal way.
5 At some stage take further X-rays to prove all foreign bodies have been removed if dealing with multiple foreign bodies.

Skin markers over wound
held with sellotape

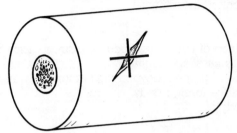

Two X-rays required
in two planes at
right-angles

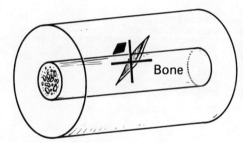

Foreign body
on antero-posterior
view approximate
site located

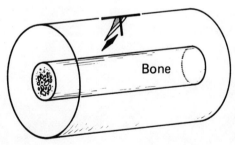

Foreign body
on lateral view
This gives an
indication of depth

91 Nose

For the removal of foreign bodies from the nose, usually in children.

A Good light source and head mirror (*see page 206*)
B A suitable blunt hooked instrument
C Nasal speculum

1 Confirm the presence of the foreign body by direct vision using the head mirror and nasal speculum.
2 Pass the hook of the instrument beyond the foreign body and turn the hook to contact the foreign body.
3 Pull the foreign body out.

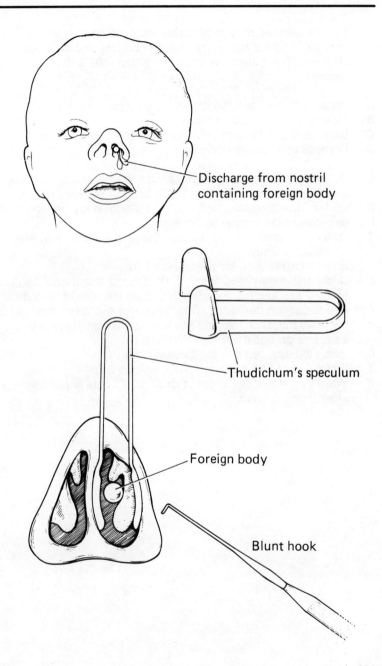

Discharge from nostril containing foreign body

Thudichum's speculum

Foreign body

Blunt hook

For the removal of foreign bodies from the back of the oral cavity and the oropharynx. Some foreign bodies will show on X-ray. However the patient is the best judge that a foreign body is present.

A   Suitable spray anaesthetic (10 per cent cocaine)
B   Head mirror and light source
C   Laryngeal mirrors and methylated lamp
D   Forceps and tongue depressor

1   Sit yourself down comfortably facing the patient, so that you can use the head mirror to direct light into the patient's mouth.
2   Under direct vision look for a foreign body in the mouth, depressing the tongue as necessary.
3   Spray the back of the mouth and oropharynx with the local anaesthetic spray.
4   Have a further look for the foreign body.
5   Using the methylated lamp, heat a laryngeal mirror slightly to prevent misting, but not enough to burn the patient. Introduce the mirror through the mouth. Turn the mirror and direct the light from the head mirror so that you can see a reflection of the larynx. Look for a foreign body.
6   Using forceps, remove the foreign body.
7   If you do not find a foreign body, ask for help.
8   Warn the patient not to eat or drink for 2 hours to permit the local anaesthetic to wear off.

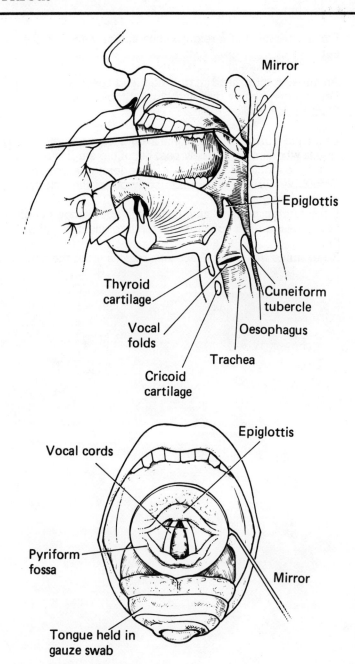

Mirror

Epiglottis

Thyroid cartilage

Cuneiform tubercle

Vocal folds

Oesophagus

Trachea

Cricoid cartilage

Vocal cords

Epiglottis

Pyriform fossa

Mirror

Tongue held in gauze swab

93 Ears

For the removal of foreign bodies and/or wax from the external ear.

A An auriscope (or head mirror, light and specula)
B Ear syringe, kidney dish and bowl of tepid water
C Blunt hook

1 Using the auriscope check the nature of the foreign body, and assess whether it will freely pass out of the ear if syringed. Check that the patient has no history of a perforated eardrum.
2 If possible syringe the foreign body out of the external acoustic meatus (*see page 208*).
3 If the foreign body is such that it will not syringe out of the ear, gently pass a blunt hook beyond the foreign body and pull it out of the ear.
4 Re-examine the external acoustic meatus using the auriscope.

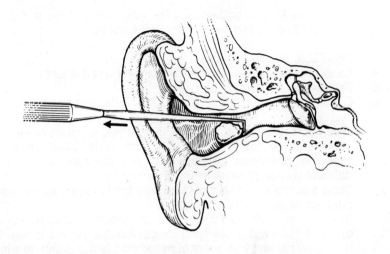

To remove foreign bodies from the conjunctiva or the surface of the cornea, including the conjunctival fornices.

A Good light source
B Local anaesthetic eye drops (1.0 per cent amethocaine)
C Fluorescein eye drops
D Cotton wool buds, orange sticks, 25G needle and small syringe

1 With good illumination examine the cornea, conjunctiva and the fornices of the conjunctiva for a foreign body. Evert the upper eyelid as described on *page 202.* Ask the patient to look in different directions to assist the examination.
2 Using a cotton wool bud it may be possible to wipe a foreign body from the surface of the conjunctiva.
3 If the foreign body is on the cornea, anaesthetize the surface of the eye with the local anaesthetic drops. Ask the patient to turn his face upwards and look away from the side (left or right) on which the foreign body is present. Put two drops of anaesthetic in the lateral corner of the eye.
4 Try wiping the foreign body from the cornea with a cotton wool bud. If this fails then use a 25G needle (on a small syringe as holder) to pick the foreign body from the surface of the cornea. Do not dig into the cornea.
5 Stain the eye with the fluorescein drops and examine the cornea under a bluish light for any signs of ulceration. If a corneal ulcer is present ask for specialist help.
6 If you have used local anaesthetic drops then apply a pad to the eye for protection until the anaesthetic effect wears off.

94 Eyes

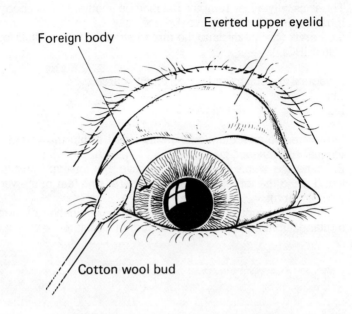

Foreign body

Everted upper eyelid

Cotton wool bud

95 Vagina

This is usually a lost Tampax, but may be another foreign body. An Intra-Uterine Contraceptive Device may be presenting through the cervix (do not mistake the thread attached to the IUCD for the actual IUCD).

A   A vaginal speculum and a good light source.
B   Ring forceps
C   Lubricating jelly and gloves

1   Lubricate the speculum and gently insert it into the vagina (*see vaginal examination page 130*).
2   Examine the whole vagina and remove any foreign body that is found using the forceps. Check that there is no tear of the vaginal wall or cervix.
3   Remove the speculum and complete the examination by doing a digital examination of the vagina, and an abdominal examination.

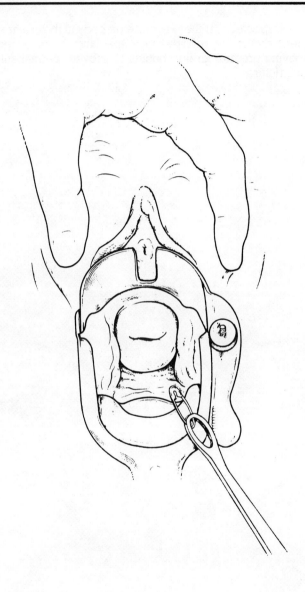

If it is suspected that there is a foreign body in the urethra, then the patient should be referred to a specialist. Care is required in removing urethral foreign bodies to prevent permanent damage and stricture.

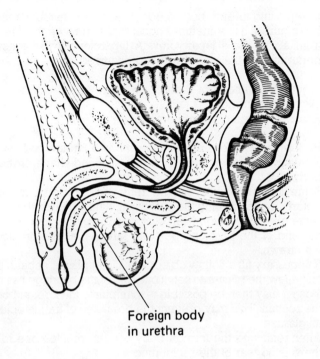

Foreign body
in urethra

97 Rectum

In removing foreign bodies from the rectum, much ingenuity may be required. It is sometimes necessary to remove the foreign body from above via a laparotomy. A laparotomy will be essential if perforation of the bowel wall has occurred.

A   Proctoscope and light source
B   Gloves and lubricating jelly
C   Assorted instruments and other agents

1   Perform a rectal examination to confirm a foreign body is present.
2   X-rays of the pelvis may show the size and shape of the foreign body.
3   Some foreign bodies can be removed by digital manipulation, before or after dilating the anal canal. It may be possible to remove some objects through a proctoscope, or by holding them against the end of the proctoscope (with forceps) as the proctoscope is withdrawn.
4   If necessary fill a hollow object with a wet plaster of paris bandage and allow the plaster to set. If one end of the bandage has been left loose it may then be possible to manipulate the foreign body out of the rectum. This may prevent the breakage of fragile objects such as glasses.
5   After removing the foreign body use the proctoscope to confirm there is no tear of the rectal mucosa.

Foreign body in rectum

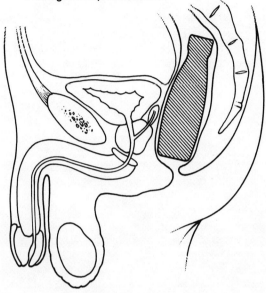

Foreign body shown on X-ray

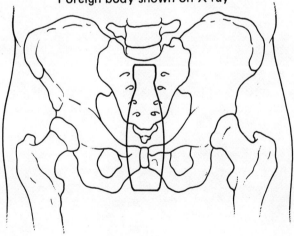

Index

235